Corona

and the

Human Heart

Corona
and the
Human Heart

Illuminating riddles of
immunity, conscience and
common sense

Dr Michaela Glöckler

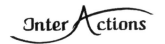

First published in German as
Das Herz als Zentralorgan des Immunsystems,
Ort des Gewissens und des gesunden Menschenverstand,
a section in
Corona und das Rätsel der Immunität,
Akanthos Akademie Edition, 2nd Edition 2021

Original German text amended and updated
by the author and publisher for the English edition.
Translation by
Gaby Horsley

First published in English by
InterActions 2021

ISBN 978-0-9528364-5-2

Layout by InterActions
Printed in the UK
by ImprintDigital.com

Contents

Foreword

I would like to express my gratitude to the publishers of Inter-Actions for taking the initiative to make this manuscript available to the readers at this critical time of rampant anxiety and growing mistrust towards an increasingly dogmatic and authoritarian use of science. When I first came across this text, as a chapter in the comprehensive, multi-author book "Corona and the Riddle of Immunity,"[1] edited by Michaela Glöckler and Andreas Neider, I was struck by its unique perspective that goes well beyond the proverbial focus on disease and its methods of eradication.

As we make way well into the second year of the pandemic and are faced with the emergence of new, seemingly more aggressive variants of the virus that are spreading even in countries where draconian lockdowns, quarantines and travel restrictions were enforced from early on, one wonders whether resorting to such measures was effective in the first place? Given that "breakthrough" Covid-19 cases occur amongst individuals who chose or were coerced into accepting the still experimental "vaccines," it is reasonable to ask whether the promotion of measures that strengthen resilience and natural immunity would have been a better choice? Short of promoting global vaccination mandates, the World Health Organization, govern-

---

[1] Corona und das Rätsel der Immunität, edited by Michaela Glöckler and Andreas Neider, Stuttgart: Akanthos Akademie, *2nd edition 2021. Not yet published in English.*

ments, and public health agencies appear to be running out of options in their efforts to limit the spread. Captivated by the alleged effectiveness of the "Chinese model," some politicians and health officials now subscribe to the enforcement of digital contact tracing and vaccination passports. These and other such measures not only deny personal autonomy but eerily resemble methods used by surveillance states, the infrastructure for which already exists in form of electronic media.

In the face of numerous historical precedents, one wonders, what happened to common sense? It is remarkable to witness how individual rights and medical freedom, guaranteed by the constitution and international conventions, can evaporate into thin air and be superseded by mandates and emergency decrees in the name of "safety for all." As foreseen by some, and in hindsight acknowledged by many others, it is becoming clear how rigorously enforced lockdowns and isolation measures erode psychological as well as physical well-being of a vast majority of the population that was spared the illness or suffered only a relatively mild form. The fact that repetitive stress, fear, and insecurity weaken immunity and predispose to ill health has been amply documented in the research literature ranging from psychoneuroimmunology to neurocardiology. However, the real nature of the psychic-bodily interaction remains an open question.

Despite being the subject of perennial discussion within the ranks of academic medicine and psychology, the brain/mind dichotomy, also known as the "Cartesian duality" remains at the level of a hypothesis, an intellectual construct with little prospect of being solved. For the materialistically minded, ideas, purpose, meaning, joy of life, grief, friendship, and love are simply emanations of the neurons within the brain. This view is contested by those who believe that consciousness can exist independently of matter, a sort of mind-stuff composed of non-material substantiality, as confirmed by numerous reports of near-death and end-of-life experiences. The origins of this separation can be traced to the atomists in ancient Greece, beginning with Democritus and his followers and has since been elevated to the status of a scientific dogma. It gained momentum with the 17th century positivist thinkers for whom only the outer, material phenomena that could be measured, weighed, or quantified in any way, were considered objective and real, whereas sensations such as sound, smell, taste, or warmth were deemed to be merely subjective experiences, bereft of reality. The discovery, that there is no substantial difference between the physical and chemical components of the human organism and those of the mineral realm into which the body disintegrates after death, led to the assumption that matter is the primary principle of existence and life and its myriad manifestations only its derivative, an epiphenomenon. Similarly, neuroscientists assume that consciousness is only a complicated form of material processes that can be explained solely by neuronal activity. Given that neurobiological processes in humans and higher primates are remarkably similar, it is hardly surprising that a human being is considered merely a "higher animal." By reducing the human being to "biological machinery," medicine has obliterated in content as well as by method what is experienced, felt, and suffered in dimensions of life, feelings, and thoughts – in short, what makes a human being human.

Dr Glöckler informs us that the "Cartesian duality" has, in fact, been bridged by a line of ontological idealist thinkers who foresaw the dire consequences of science and medicine based on reductionist assumptions. They made – and continue to make, as exemplified by this contribution – pioneering efforts to expand the method of science to encompass not only the physical-material aspect of nature, but also the living and the sentient. Finally, we owe it to Rudolf Steiner, who systematically addressed the fundamental question of scientific methodology in his ground-breaking epistemological writings. He laid the foundation for a new, participatory way of science derived from methods first described by Goethe. Steiner's revolutionary breakthrough was to characterize the human as a multidimensional being consisting of four levels of organization, namely, of the physical body, the life or etheric body, and of soul and spirit.

Fully cognizant of the limitations of the conventional approach, Dr Glöckler explores the question of immunity from the Goethean perspective and discovers a striking reciprocity between the biological and the spiritual resilience or immunity. The former is an expression of our Self, which impresses its unique "stamp of identity" on every organ and cell of the body. This gives rise to the so-called tissue and humoral immunity which protects us from everything that is foreign or "not-self," be it microorganisms, allergens, or antigens. The opposite is the case in the domain of the soul where moral qualities and virtues shine brightest when egotism is transformed into selflessness and altruism. The author shows us how the highest member of the human organization, the ego, manifests itself organically as well as psychically, much alike the Roman god of gates, Janus, represented by a double-faced head looking in opposite directions. Remarkably, the place of this crucial transformation is none other than the human heart!

This timely book represents a breakthrough in phenomenological research that will provide far-reaching insights not only to those who are prompted by the current pandemic to ask deeper questions related to health and medical freedom, but also to all open-minded researchers in pursuit of bridging the mind-body divide.

Branko Furst, MD
Kinderhook, New York
July 2021

Introduction

'This pandemic harms interests, affects biographies and jeopardises livelihoods. There are no unobjectionable decisions at this present time' said Gabor Steingart in his morning briefing on 19th November 2020. It was the day after the German government had ratified the 3rd amendment to the Infection Control Act, with 415 votes in favour, 236 against and 8 abstentions. This Act severely restricts the fundamental rights and freedom of the individual. Countless livelihoods are at risk. Internationally, hunger and poverty become unbearable, the refugee crisis is escalating, and fear and aggression are omnipresent. Every day we are presented with the latest numbers of infections and the danger that, even if there are sufficient Intensive Care Unit (ICU) beds, there may not be enough nursing staff to look after the patients. As of summer 2021 not much has changed. Now the news is full of reports of virus mutations.

Society is polarising on all levels, reaching into families, work teams and work contexts. Communication between 'scaremongers' and 'Covidiots'[2] is hardly possible. On top of that, the 'Covidiots' fear that they are seen as right-wing extremists or as conspiracy theorists. How can mediation succeed in such a climate? Which authority can I turn to in the face of the daily barrage of news shown by media and on the internet presenting contradictory opinions and information?

With all this going on, is there any place for common sense?

---

[2]   'Covidiots' is a term used in British press; 'Covid sceptics' is more common in USA.

Are we now dependent only on the latest scientific insights and their inconsistencies? Where do I stand? How do I not only maintain my own judgement but even develop it further in view of the media announcements and many a critical voice from the ranks of committed medical professionals and contemporaries who dare to speak up? What does my voice of conscience say? How do I regain my optimism and my confidence? Where are the wellsprings of courage, mental and emotional health and trust? How can I work on my health potential and contribute constructively to the complex consequences of this pandemic?

More and more people are unsure how humanity will manage all the potential perils, wondering what life will be like in 10 years' time: will it be a global surveillance state, where safety is more valued than the risk of a life in freedom? Will humanity be able to use modern technologies in service of cultural evolution or will it become more and more dependent on them? Mario Vargas Llosa, the Nobel prize winner for literature said in an interview with Neue Zürcher Zeitung (a Swiss newspaper) dated 2nd November 2020: 'The fine line between sensible measures to contain the pandemic and usurpation of power politics is naturally very narrow … And if we lose this freedom, we lose everything in the long run. Without it, all is nothing.' What does our heart say to all of this? What message does our voice of conscience have? Is there such a thing as common sense? And is there such a thing as 'medical' common sense?

How do we recognise common sense and how can we cultivate it?

What characterises common sense?

'Healthy' common sense is based on a concern for the truth and the love of life. Because facts are one thing, and their interpretation and consequences for daily life are another. A prominent example is the PCR test. Its presumed validity forms the basis for the entire strategy of track-and-trace and the consequences of the lockdown.[3] The daily figures of the Robert-Koch-Institute as well as from other countries have shown that around 20% of those who tested positive do not develop any symptoms and are therefore not contagious.[4] Contagiosity is based on symptoms. Only if the virus can become virulent – which is causing mild or severe symptoms, is it possible to spread it. Nevertheless, because of the eventual risk that one could develop symptoms

---

[3]   This book does not examine further questions around the PCR test, for example: how significant are the (positive PCR tested) case numbers if the tests are carried out to a Ct value of >35 (as most currently are)? The reader is referred to Dr Thomas Hardtmuth's book, *What Covid-19 Can Teach Us* (InterActions, 2021), for an in-depth discussion.

[4]   See https://www.meinbezirk.at/niederoesterreich/c-regionauten-community/corona-positiv-getestet-aber-symptomlos-krankheit-oder-immunitaet_a4154610 [Corona positive test but without symptoms – illness or immunity?] and https://www.tt.com/artikel/17415771/ein-viertel-der-positiv-auf-corona-getesten-nicht-infektioes [A quarter of those testing positive for Corona not infectious]

in the days to come, one has to self-isolate. Fortunately this is mostly not happening, but the insecurity remains as a problem. We have no clear numbers for how many of those asymptomatic but positive tested people are later showing symptoms – the studies have not been organised! Indications so far are that it is small. All positive tested, with and without symptoms, are seen as 'healed' after quarantine. About 80% of infected people develop mostly mild symptoms, and a few people develop severe symptoms; according to the WHO, by 18th August 2021, 2.4% of the 3.8 million people infected with Corona in Germany had died of or with it. So, 97.6% of infected people recover or even stay well without developing the illness at all.

Given these figures, is not the risk of falling severely from Covid quite low for people under 70 and those not having special pre-existing conditions? Is it not the fear-mongering and the reports of terrible individual cases that make me fearful so that I conclude 'better err on the side of caution'? Facts are one thing, how we interpret them is another. This also applies to exponential calculations. For example, it is a well-known fact that a baby doubles its birth weight within the first five months. However, it would be irrelevant to ask: how heavy will the child therefore be in three years' time? Of course, we can calculate that – but it does not match the reality of life. Thinking and calculations may be fact-based and logical, and yet be incorrect in regard to real life.

Common Sense is firmly rooted in the reality of life and never views facts in isolation but rather in context - including that of personal life experiences. This creates inner certainty which allows us to stand by our viewpoint, even if it does not coincide with any of the mainstream views. For illustration, here are five examples:

1. A teacher discusses with her colleagues and the parents and pupils of her class the real-life risks of wearing masks in the classroom. Even with the best ventilation of the room everybody in the classroom breathes the same air which contains a certain number of viruses (not just Corona virus!). Although the masks are effective in preventing the distribution of droplets, fine aerosols still escape through the holes at the edges of the mask where the air moves faster than through the fabric of the mask. Everyone can check that for themselves using their own mask.

There is no doubt that masks help to reduce the viral load, but inevitably everyone in the classroom breathes the same air, especially as the students and teachers are together every day, just like family units. In that way the class forms a so-called cluster – in other words a virus community.

Can we not agree to carry the remaining risk together, to conduct normal lessons and do away with the requirement to wear masks in the classroom? Of course, only if everyone agrees. This could be discussed with the local authorities, supported by official comparisons with other classes where those involved want to comply with the mask requirement and decide to forgo singing.

What is the relative benefit of a relaxed, pleasant and normal lesson experience compared to the potential harm of the whole class having to quarantine for 5 or even 10 days if one of the children tests positive? What speaks against such 'controlled freedom', given that children rarely infect adults, children's symptoms are usually mild and there has been no case of pneumonia to date? Such an approach adapted to the reality of life has the advantage that people speak to and respect each other and find a consensus which everyone can agree to. And for many people the anxiety level will go down when they learn about resilience factors and strategies to strengthen the immune system. Children need to be seen and protected – adults can protect themselves.

2. The majority of parents in a Waldorf kindergarten request that the teacher work with the children in the normal, familiar way without wearing a mask. The parents of one child disagree and threaten to report the teacher. It is possible to settle this dispute amicably with the parents agreeing that they will register their child in another local kindergarten. A win-win situation can be established by using common sense and respecting everyone's needs.

3. Stephan Seiler reports on 18th November 2020 in the Newsletter of 'Corona Transition': 'Exceptionally high excess mortality in Switzerland'. This was the headline in the Tagesanzeiger (a Swiss daily newspaper) on 17th November. It said, the number of deaths of the over-65-year-olds had risen dramatically between 2nd and 8th November (week 45) compared to the long-term average for the same week. Swissinfo, the international broadcast of the Swiss radio and television agency (Schweizer Radio- und Fernsehgesellschaft), also ran the headline: 'Second Covid wave leads to increased number of excess deaths.'

Seiler states, 'I wanted to know more detail and analysed the data provided by the Federal Statistical Office. Result: Indeed, in week 45 of 2020, 507 more people died than the average of the previous 5 years – after all, an increase of 36%. But – and this is very important – such weekly variations are normal and in no way representative. When one compares the number of deaths of over-65-year-olds in week 41 with the 5 year average the figures looked quite different: 59 more deaths in the over 65s – an increase of 5.2% over the 5-year average. This is roughly seven times less than figures given by Tagesanzeiger and Swissinfo who chose week 45. In week 35 of 2020 there were even 105 fewer deaths compared to the last 5 years.'

The chart below (Figure 1a) shows how the death figures for Switzerland up until summer 2021 have fluctuated over the past few years and how a statistic given for any one particular week will invariably not be representative of the broader picture. (The Z-score shown is a measure of deviation from normal rather than an absolute figure of deaths.) For interpretations, it is also helpful to see actual death figures in the context of seasonal variations, as Figure 1b shows for European countries.

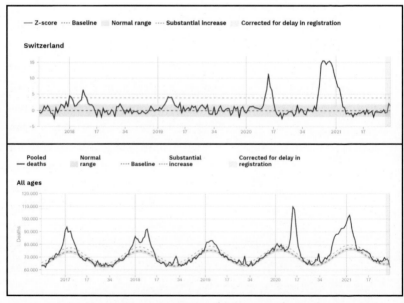

Source: from www.euromomo.eu/graphs-and-maps

Figures 1a and 1b – Deaths as deviation from normal in Switzerland, and seasonal pattern of total deaths within European countries.

So, instead of immediately reacting to the fear-driven headlines, is it not better to 'pause', reflect and investigate what other factors need to be considered? For example, by looking at Figure 1b, charting fatalities over several years, we can realise that not all deaths in the recorded recent 'waves' are out of the ordinary. We may be prompted then to research further. The approach is similar to not immediately passing judgement on someone on the basis of an unpleasant observation – if we try to understand why someone might behave in a certain way we have an entirely different relationship to them. This has a self-empowering effect, and we can have the conviction of 'owning' our responses. As we know in medicine, reflection and understanding further activity in the frontal cortex of the brain, a hallmark for human development, whereas merely reacting emotionally or fearfully bypasses this part of the brain, with actions based on 'fight or flight' mechanisms.

4. A similar experience to the above can be had with the current pressure around Covid vaccinations. As physicians, we have a great responsibility around the prescribing of medications, and both our training and conscience is built around the principle of *informed consent* given by the patient. We discuss with the patient the different possible treatments, and if there are any risks involved we certainly make these clear and allow the patient to make their own decision. Our experience, however, with Covid vaccines is that open discussion is being discouraged and, in the press, even censored. Some doctors and nurses fear for losing work or even being taken off the register if they raise questions. But as with all medications, the public needs to know all the information around the vaccines, from side-effects (of which there have been many reported) to alternatives. These are not being made readily available, though examination of data even in government reports shows the validity of questions raised. Discussion around preventative measures has nearly dropped

from media reporting, though any doctor or informed person will know that all we can do to stay in good health will help protect us against all manner of illnesses, including Covid. On the question of Covid vaccination of children now being promoted, parents need to be especially careful and fully informed because we do not yet know the long-term effects of mRNA vaccines in a period of life, in which the body and immune system are still in process of development. And is it justified to take the risk of a post vaccine myocarditis in childhood and youth, if it is known, that Covid in childhood is causing almost no harm and that the immunity after having had Covid is better than after vaccination?

If we take this informed consent approach seriously, we gain a new feeling of self-engagement and empowerment. Rather than (re)acting from fear, pressure or even coercion, our reflection and subsequent decisions come from our self. This makes a huge difference, because only then we can stand fully behind the decision and what might be its consequences.

5. A religion teacher shared an occurrence in one of her lessons. She asked 28 children in class 5 whether they would report their neighbours when they saw that more than two families were meeting there (at this time, the 2nd lockdown in Germany was well under way). 27 children answered yes, this must be reported. Only one child said no. Which of these answers is more compassionate and thus more appropriate to life circumstances? Which answer requires more courage and authenticity? For sure, the 27 children felt justified. But if you do not know why there were more than two families at the neighbours at that time you cannot know whether it was due to exceptional circumstances. When you judge only according to numbers and the law you lose sight of the individual, human situation. This sort of

question can spark valuable discussions about the difference between denunciation and the obligation to notify the authorities.

6. A medical colleague told me that she visited a relative in ICU who had had a heart attack. From then on, my colleague supported the patient's family. The patient died soon thereafter, and it was agreed that the family could pick up the coffin. But then they were informed at short notice that the coffin would not be released because of Covid. My colleague, acting on behalf of the family, contacted a senior staff member and asked for the reason: although the corona PCR test had been negative twice, the death certificate stated the patient as Corona positive. Because of this inconsistency, and because she was able to conduct a professional discussion, my colleague succeeded in obtaining the release of the coffin. However, the diagnosis remained unchanged: Death due to heart attack with Covid-19. Presumably, that was for financial reasons - the intensive care of a Covid-19 patient is paid more highly. My colleague commented afterwards 'this has taught me to treat the numbers which are reported from Intensive Care Units with caution. I cannot simply believe them anymore.' Law and Order is one thing – the reality of life another.

Preliminary conclusion: Common sense develops through life - for life. It is important to stay awake, to take seriously what you read and experience every day and to question things that seem odd. The more people do this and have the courage to share it, the less we need to fear the total surveillance which is currently so welcomed by the majority of people and politicians based on the notions of safety and security. In our fully digitised daily life, with its dwindling possibilities of paying cash or reading a menu and ordering food in an analogue fashion, we must recognise that privacy is becoming an alien concept. Instead, politics and economics profit from a massive increase in power due to the new flood of data which is harvested from our daily activities.

The great opportunity offered by this pandemic, however, is as obvious as the known dangers: to be even more alert to the radical changes in the political and economic arenas, realising shared responsibility for what is happening, witnessing with open eyes the great push for digital transformation and co-creating this transformation as constructively as possible.

Conditions which support the development of common sense

The above examples show that healthy common sense is not based on complacency, shallowness and focus on safety, but on the development of personal initiative, self-efficacy, honest concern and consciousness of individual freedom. However, a central educational challenge for our present time is that the free thinking, courage and risk-taking do not lead into chaos. The current educational systems are not equipped to deal with this moral challenge. Through their test culture and one-sided emphasis on performance they foster conformity and a striving for security. Being continually compared with 'better' and 'worse' pupils corrupts the development of healthy self-confidence. The 'better' performers become arrogant – the 'worse' performers become depressed.[5] Self-confidence can only develop in a healthy way when a child's progress is seen in relation to themselves, and when they experience their progress with joy. Children need educators who accompany them and who can help them learn from his mistakes. In that way, children can develop healthy self-esteem as well as tolerance of the mistakes of others. Ethics and values cannot be taught – they must be experienced and practiced from an early age so that they can become part of a person's character.

---

[5]   Compare Michaela Glöckler, *Education for the Future: How to nurture health and human potential?* Stroud: Interactions, 2020.

What is the relationship between the heart and the immune system?

Normally, we do not associate the heart with the immune system. Yet the immune system develops as an integral part of the blood. The blood, blood vessels and the heart (the central organ of the vascular system) develop as a coherent unit from very early on in the embryonic stage, that is, they share the same precursor cells – the so-called haemangioblasts. Haemangioblasts already evolve before gastrulation - at the end of the second and beginning of the third week of gestation. These stem cells provide the foundation for the formation of blood vessels, including the endocardial tubes which later give rise to the heart organ. Haemangioblasts are also the precursors of blood cells: the red blood cells (erythrocytes) which transport oxygen, and the immuno-competent white blood cells (leukocytes) which protect the organism from harmful influences.

Interestingly, the formation of blood cells and blood vessels begins almost simultaneously in the so-called embryonal sheaths - the yolk sac, the allantois, connecting stalk and chorion. As soon as the first blood vessels on the yolk sac and the allantois have differentiated, at the beginning of the third week, the formation of the blood and the blood vessels begins in the foetus itself. Small blood islands form everywhere which give rise to vessel segments and motile blood cells. The small vessel segments connect with each other to form larger vessel segments.

The blood flows inside these vessel segments. Thus the first impulse for the formation of the cardio-vascular system comes from the embryonal sheaths which the embryo forms around itself before it begins to grow.

This is the primal gesture of all living things: life is not possible without an adequate environment, surroundings which provide both support and purpose. So it is not surprising that the embryo first develops its environment or milieu before it begins to mature. From the very beginning, this primal gesture of centre and periphery forms the archetypal basis for the configuration of the cardiovascular system.

Centre and periphery develop towards each other simultaneously; neither can exist without the other. The initial yolk sac circulation, which develops early on, readily supports the embryo's nourishment and respiration using sensitive visceral perception and feedback processes which gauge the required amounts of nutrients and oxygen.

The primitive cardiac system, which is located below the head of the embryo, becomes connected to the embryonal blood vessels, and then begins to beat on day 21.[6] The latest research shows that the endothelial cells within the blood vessel tissues are 'sensors' for the metabolic demands of the tissues and integrate the flow of blood, i.e. the amount of delivered oxygen and nutrients. Through this they support the subsequently developing cardiovascular system.[7] You cannot simply see the heart as a pressure generating pump and the source of blood's move-

---

[6]   See Keith L. Moore, T.V.M. Persaud and Mark G. Torchia, *The Developing Human: Clinically Oriented Embryology,* 9th ed. New York: Saunders, 2012.

[7]   See Branko Furst, *The Heart and Circulation. An integrative Model.* Berlin: Springer Nature, 2020, p. 42.

ment if you are aware of the intricate synergy which is at play during the configuration of the heart and circulatory system. Rather you perceive the heart as a central organ which works as coordinator and initiator, surrounded by an actively pulsating and working periphery.

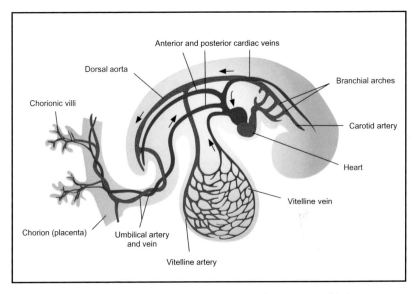

Figure 2: Schematic representation of a 26-day old embryo with its early embryonic circulation. From the chorion (precursor of the placenta) the nutrient-rich blood vessels lead through the connecting stalk (later the umbilical cord) into the embryo, and from there into the venous vessels (coloured blue) returning the oxygen-poor blood, which also contains metabolic waste products, to the chorion.

It is amazing that all the various specialised cells - which form the blood, the blood vessels with their smooth muscles and the heart itself with its specialised cardiac muscle structure - have got *one* common type of precursor cell: the cardiovascular progenitor cell or the hemangioblast.

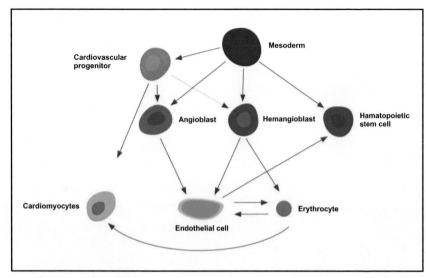

Figure 3. This illustration shows the pluripotent mesoderm cell, the origin of all cells which form the blood and the blood-vessels. The mesodermal cells form the so-called middle cotyledon, which is generated in the third week of embryonic development between the outer cotyledon (progenitor) and the inner cotyledon (endoderm). The arrows indicate the respective origins of the cells.

The blood requirement increases continuously from the 2nd month onward. After the chorion, as the most important place of blood formation in the first weeks, the intensive haematopoietic activity continues in the liver, which in week 9 constitutes 10% of the total body weight of the embryo. Later on, the spleen and finally the bone marrow take over the blood production together with the developing lymph nodes, and the hematopoietic activity in the liver ceases. All these organs are capable of forming blood stem cells as precursors for the red blood cells and the abundance of differentiated immune-competent white cells. The lymphatic system is exceptional in so far as it begins to emerge only from week 5, about two weeks later than the vascular system, because precursor cells for this system grow out of endothelial outgrowths from veins and are oriented towards immunological functions from the outset.[8]

The cardiovascular system is the first functioning organ system in the embryo – already at the end of the third week the blood begins to circulate and the heart begins to beat. It is the organ system that accompanies the entire embryonic development and which up until the very end continues to develop in full resonance with it. The final point of this process is reached after birth when the foetal circulation is terminated and the independent circulation of the new-born infant begins, connected to the lungs and the external air. During the embryonic and foetal development no organ is able to form and mature without the permeation of blood vessels stimulating growth processes and ensuring the supply of necessary nutrients as well as the removal of waste products.

The 'fluid organ structure' of the blood-lymph-system works in three main areas:

• The red blood cells together with endothelial cells which line the blood vessels act as 'mobile sensors' by monitoring the oxygen demand - not only in the lungs but also at the tissue level of the entire organism. Thereby they regulate the oxygen supply to all the tissues according to need.

• The red blood cells serve for the transport of oxygen and the absorption of carbon dioxide, the blood plasma for the transport and distribution of nutrients.

• The so-called white blood cells (lymphocytes – normally between 20 to 50% of total while cells – and leukocytes) guard against viruses, bacteria and harmful substances. They serve as general protection against harmful influences

---

8   Ibid, p. 75.

together with other barrier functions of the body, such as the skin.

Three particular types of protective function were discussed widely in connection with the Corona pandemic:

- The non-specific innate immunity. It facilitates a wide range of sensitivity to bacteria and viruses and ensures that some people 'are never sick'. It is also due to the non-specific immunity that some groups of people, even entire countries, saw only very few serious Covid cases. This is down to the spectrum of immunomodulators and complement factors which are released into the blood plasma; and also white blood cells (e.g. various granulocytes such as neutrophils and eosinophils, as well as monocytes, which specialise in rendering harmful substances and pathogens harmless).

- The specific, so-called adaptive competence of the immune system. This is based on the recognition of antigens and the subsequent activation of B-lymphocytes which can form antibodies within 5-7 days.

- The so-called T lymphocytes.[9] These can form surface T-cell receptors (TCRs) for the purpose of binding specific antigens which are related to certain pathogens.[10]

---

[9]   T and B cells refer to tissue and blood cell immunity, respectively.
[10]   See Peter Vaupel, Hans-Georg Schaible and Ernst Mutschler, Anatomie, Physiologie, Pathophysiologie des Menschen [Human anatomy, physiology, pathophysiology]. 7th completely revised and enlarged edition. Stuttgart: Wissenschafliche Verlagsgesellschaft, 2015, p. 177.

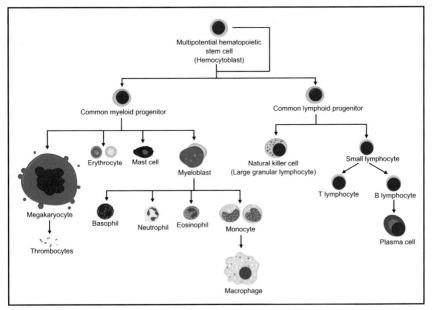

Figure 4: This diagram shows the profusion of the various red and white blood cells and their common origin in the stem cell population capable of giving rise to all these different configurations. It also illustrates that the specific defence cells of the lymphatic system – the so-called T cells, natural killer cells and B cells – are formed from the same stem cell type as the red and white blood cells.

Central to this whole development is the heart which itself is created through the middle cotyledon and the blood stem cells or hemangioblasts. The blood from all the regions and organs of the body converges in the heart, carrying information about the blood and lymph systems. Whereas the blood circulates in a closed circuit this is not the case with the lymph. Lymphatic capillaries begin like the blind ends of myriads of capillaries in the periphery of the body where they absorb interstitial fluid which becomes lymph in the capillaries.

Lympha in Latin means 'clear water'. The lymph can absorb nutrients as well as harmful substances or tumour cells and pathogens, rendering them harmless in the lymph nodes, before they then enter the superior vena cava via their largest collecting vessel, the thoracic duct, which ends in the right atrium of the heart. From there all the venous blood goes to the right ventricle and from there to the lungs where it absorbs oxygen. The oxygenated blood flows as arterial blood via the left atrium into the left ventricle.

Both ventricles together produce the so-called heartbeat with the associated pulse wave, which then spreads synchronously over the entire arterial system. At rest, the heart beats on average 70 times per minute and ejects 140 ml of blood (70 ml per ventricle). At a certain point during cardiac contraction and relaxation (systole and diastole) something remarkable happens which is normally overlooked: At the end of the filling phase (diastole) and before the start of the expulsion of the blood (systole) there is a moment of transition when pressure and volume remain constant for a short time; the otherwise constantly flowing blood comes to a halt for a fraction of a second.[11] Each unit of blood comes to rest in the heart at the end of the inflow before it is then expelled in the reverse direction by ventricular contraction. That special moment of transition from movement to rest and from rest to movement is of great importance for what we will consider in further sections of this book, which is why it is mentioned here. This moment of temporary rest of the blood is called diastasis in cardiac physiology.

---

[11]   The FORWARD FLOW of blood is interrupted for a fraction of a second; but the blood continues to move vortex-like within the ventricles even when the aortic and mitral valves are closed (diastasis). It is on account of these RHYTHMIC interruptions of forward flow that the heart becomes a SENSE ORGAN. A sleeping state, characterized by continuous (etheric) flow is interrupted by the breath which brings in soul-spirit, i.e., consciousness; the astral in animal and the Spirit or Self in human - on account of the upright stance.

How can we strengthen the immune system?

Spirit triumphant
Flame through the weakness
Of faint-hearted souls,
Consume their self-seeking,
Ignite their compassion,
That selflessness,
The lifestream of humankind,
May live as wellspring
Of spirit rebirth.

Rudolf Steiner

Why is selflessness the lifestream of humanity? How are protection and self-defence (immune system) related to selflessness? How does spiritual immunity differ from physical and emotional immunity? When we look at the human organism in terms of physical, emotional and spiritual activity we find a striking polarity.

Healthy digestion means that the ingested food is completely destroyed, the immune system recognising and eliminating harmful substances, so that the remaining nutritional elements can serve as building blocks for ones *own* body. Proteins which are specifically human are called the 'biological ego'.

In contrast, human mental activities (perception, thinking) can be said to work the other way round. Effective perception adapts itself to the perceived object and tries to 'grasp' it, and thus avoids falling prey to illusion. The better the perceiving and processing mind manages to comprehend objectively what is going on, the healthier it is. It is like reversed digestion – in the process of understanding I mentally 'become the other'. For example, when I want to think 'two plus two is four' I must put my thinking in the service of this mathematical task; – and I know that two plus two is not five even if this might be more amusing. We can speak of a mental or spiritual 'communion' – we become one with the object of our cognition.

The nutritional substances provided by nature must submit to complete destruction through the metabolic processes. Nature has to become human, so to speak. The opposite is true when we are searching for the truth. In the emotional life we speak of empathy when someone is able to really resonate with another's sorrow and joy. If we, instead, project our own sympathies and antipathies onto the other person, we experience ourselves rather than what is alive for them. So, selflessness results in good mental health and social competency in our soul life. On the physical level, however, selflessness would cause serious illness and the breakdown of the immune system. While biological egoism is healthy and unconsciously controlled by nature, we have to actively manage our cognitive processes by deciding where we want to focus our attention. We also have to learn to moderate our view point in the service of gaining thorough and extensive understanding.

Biological egoism proves to be advantageous for our health, whilst mental and emotional egoism causes dis-ease. Altruism in soul and spirit equals good mental health, whereas a lack of biological self-interest leads to immunological incompetence, i.e. illness.

Furthermore, thoughts and feelings have a strong influence on our state of health. This has been established by modern health research, also known as 'resilience and salutogenetic research'. Much of this knowledge is now used in the practice of psychosomatic medicine, positive psychotherapy, developmental psychology, curative education and pedagogy. The science of psycho-neuroimmunology produces ever growing evidence of how positive feelings, understanding and enthusiasm strengthen the immune system, while negative feelings such as fear, worry, constant stress, uncertainty and doubt weaken the immune system and make us more vulnerable to disease.

So it is all the more surprising that these matters were hardly discussed during the first six months of the Corona-pandemic. Furthermore, the scientists who were responsible for advising the governments did not insist on inviting input from experts in the above-mentioned fields when discussing the strategies to fight the pandemic. Let us ask some very pertinent questions: Why did the media not insist on pointing out, again and again, the wealth of already exisiting scientific and practical knowledge? Why did they not regularly publish quotes, research findings and reports which would create positive feelings and encouragement? And why not draw attention to the publications by representatives of the above listed specialist areas such as, in Germany, professors Gerald Huether, Thomas Fuchs and Remo Largo? [12] Further examples could be given.

---

[12]   See Gerald Hüther, Würde: *Was uns stark macht - als Einzelne und als Gesellschaft* [Dignity: What makes us strong – as individuals and as a society], Munich: Knaus, 2018; Thomas Fuchs, *Das Gehirn - ein Beziehungsorgan* [The Brain – an organ of relationship]. Stuttgart: Kohlhammer, 2008; Thomas Fuchs, *Ecology of the Brain: The phenomenology and biology of the*

Instead, fear, insecurity and a mood of panic were stirred up and are being continuously disseminated to this day. And yet psychology tells us how fear narrows the awareness and promotes tunnel vision focussing on a perceived threat, thereby weakening the immune system.[13]

The media were dominated by ever new case calculations (whose correlation with reality is viewed very differently even amongst experts), the hope for vaccination as the only way out of the crisis, hygiene rules, track-and-trace as well as dramatic stories of individual cases.[14] Medical systems using holistic or integrative methods were, and still are, not taken into account. Yet these treatment modalities in particular provide encouraging perspectives by integrating results of health research and spiritual aspects with mainstream medicine.

But the Corona pandemic has also made us aware of many inconsistencies which can inspire real-life thinking. For example, at the beginning of the pandemic, when faced with the first

---

embodied mind. Oxford University Press, 2018. Available online at https://oxfordmedicine.com/view/10.1093/med/9780199646883.001.0001/med-9780199646883; Thomas Fuchs, *The Brain — A Mediating Organ*, online at https://www.academia.edu/11500365/The_Brain_A_Mediating_Organ;

Remo Largo, *Zusammen leben. Das Fit-Prinzip für Gemeinschaft, Gesellschaft und Natur* [Living together. A workable principle for community, society and nature).Frankfurt am Main: S. Fischer, 2020.

[13]   See Gerald Hüther, *Biologie der Angst* [Biology of fear]. 13th edition. Vandenhoeck und Ruprecht, 2016; Thomas Fuchs, *Die Enge des Lebens. Zur Phänomenologie und Typologie der Angst.*In: H. Lang and G. Pagel, editors, *Angst und Zwang* [Fear and Compulsion]. Würzburg: Königshausen und Neumann, 2019, pp. 11-25; Michaela Glöckler, *Vom Umgang mit der Angst* [Dealing with fear] 2nd edition, Stuttgart: Urachhaus, 1993.

[14]   Laura Dodsworth's new book, *A State of Fear* (Pinter & Martin, London, 2021), documents how the British as well as other governments have 'weaponised' fear for gaining public compliance with policies, using research and experience of and employing behavioural scientists.

lockdown, it was widely agreed that hospitals should receive financial support for the provision of additional beds on ICUs and wards for Covid-19 patients. Over many years the hospital system had been run according to the profit-making principles of corporate enterprises. Many local hospitals were consequently closed down because they were no longer profitable. Due to the rationalisation measures and insufficient funding the great shortage of care personnel has not decreased but increased. Is not the real problem the egoistic, profit-oriented approach to patient care? The health service should be able to cope with recurring peak demands in times of greater need, with Covid-19 not being the first time. A life-related, altruistic approach would have immediately made intensive preparations following the first outbreaks in order to financially regenerate the health care system so that it would be prepared for potential successive waves. This would include generous grants for the training of nurses and intensive care personnel.

Investments are also needed to support high risk patients and vulnerable population groups. This includes sufficient stock of PPE (personal protection equipment) so that the sick do not need to be left alone and care homes can have appropriate visiting times. Instead of spreading fear and horror it would have been much better to educate people about the function of the immune system and how to strengthen it. This would have raised the population's awareness of their personal responsibility for their own health.

An illustration of such teaching was given by Paracelsus (1493/94 -1541), who was the most influential integrative physician at the beginning of modern history.[15]

---

[15]   See Gunhild Poerksen (ed.), *Paracelsus. Der andere Arzt - Das Buch Paragranum* [Paracelsus. A physician with a difference]. Frankfurt am Main: Fischer, 2015.

In his *Volumen Paramirum* six physicians discuss the causes of the death of a cholera patient. In this dialogue Paracelsus elucidates the fact that an illness is not caused by infection alone but also by the organism's susceptibility to be infected due to a variety of causes. This is in accord with today's knowledge about pathogen exposure and an organism's predisposition for getting infected.

The first doctor begins the dialogue by saying that the deceased had died of putrid water (The cholera bacillus was not yet known in Paracelsus' time). The second physician contradicts this by stating that everyone would have had to have died who had drunk of the foul water. This, however, was not the case. The majority had not fallen ill, and of those who had developed symptoms only some had died. The third physician speaks up at this point. He draws attention to the connection between body and soul and explains that the self-healing powers depend to a great extent on emotional well-being. The deceased had died due to his negative outlook on life. The fourth medic emphasises this by saying that a positive attitude in life depends on personality and character. The deceased must have felt dispirited, causing his death. The fifth doctor pronounces quietly: 'Dear colleagues, I had a look at his horoscope – his time had run out. Our skills are no measure for God's will.'

Now, all five physicians look expectantly towards the sixth physician to hear what he might contribute. Paracelsus has him say that all five are correct – there are five gateways to illness, and also five gateways to health. A physician with sound medical intuition serves life to the end by establishing what is needed to strengthen the quality of life and the resources for each patient's health.[16]

---

16 Willem F. Daems, Paracelsus: *Die okkulten Ursachen der Krankheiten*

Anthroposophic medicine also works with these five aspects. It will be interesting to view the data of ICUs once the Corona crisis has ended. It was gratifying to hear that not a single ICU patient had died in the anthroposophic hospital Havelhoehe by October 2020 - despite high numbers of patients - as this hospital was one of the first Corona emergency units in Berlin at the beginning of the pandemic.[17]

This positive outcome was not only due to the integrative approach with its medicinal preparations and the physiological treatment of high temperature, which takes into account that fever stimulates the immune system and aids the neutralisation of viruses. It was also crucial that relatives were able to visit the patients in the ICU (with relevant PPE) from the outset. This social contact gave patients hope and confidence.

We can currently only speculate that pandemic anxiety, fears, uncertainty, worries and doubts gripping people of all ages have cost even more lives than the virus. Hopefully this will be the subject of thorough retrospective research so that we can be better prepared for future pandemics.

Physical Aspects of Immunity

A strong physical immune system is passed on to babies born into a family whose members are usually healthy, i.e. who have a strong innate basic immunity. Clinical immunology distinguishes hereditary from adaptive immune competence (as explained above). Inherent immune competence, which can affect whole ethnic groups, is seen by experts as one of the main rea-

[Occult causes of illnesses]. In: *Volumen Paramirum*. 4th edition. Dornach: Verlag am Goetheanum, 1991.

[17] See Harald Matthes, *Vom Katastrophenmodus der Politik zum risikostratifizierten Handeln* [Moving from disaster orientated politics to risk-stratified action]. Interview in: Erziehungskunst 10/2020.

sons why the Corona pandemic has had a less dramatic impact on Asian countries compared to Southern Europe and America. Adaptive immune competence, on the other hand, stems from immune adjustments which are built up from infancy through infections and vaccinations. Every mother knows that, as a rule, she does not catch infections from her child, rather, it is the adults who pass on flu viruses to their children. This is also the case with the Corona virus, though exceptions, as always, confirm the rule.

What is emotional and spiritual immunity?

Here, we enter the field of health research. I would like to illustrate this with the example of Salutogenic (= 'sources of health') research, founded by medical sociologist Aaron Antonovsky (1923-1994). He researched the state of health in older women and was surprised to find survivors of the Holocaust amongst the healthiest women.

He had suspected a particularly high post-traumatic burden as well as emotional and physical damage in Holocaust survivors. However, in reality, he found that the opposite was the case. Based on these outcomes, Antonovsky posed the question: What are the conditions under which health can get established and maintained? Based on the results of comprehensive questionnaires and accompanying interviews he identified the most important condition for good health: positive emotional connections with the people and events in one's life.

Antonovsky termed this feeling 'the sense of coherence' - of 'being part of', 'in sync with' or 'in resonance'. He discovered three specific emotional competences which are particularly health-enhancing in this context:

- The feeling of comprehensibility
- The feeling of meaningfulness or sense of purpose
- The feeling of manageability

In contrast to this, the emotional wellbeing is weakened when one no longer understands oneself and the world, when one feels misunderstood, when life or the current situation one is in feels meaningless, and when one feels powerless with the sense of 'I cannot do what I want to do' and 'I cannot be how/what I want to be'. Evidently, the women who survived the Holocaust had succeeded in meeting the extremely inhumane circumstances with inner strength.[18] [132]

The health researcher and positivist psychotherapist Abraham Maslow (1908-1970) contributed even further to the solving of this riddle. He discovered that these extraordinary people remained healthy not only due to their ability to convert negative outer experiences into positive inner experiences, they also had had spiritual experiences which Maslow terms *Peak Experience*.[19]

They found new strengths through the deep experience of a direct connection with a higher, spiritual world and of being spiritually recognised and inspired. They gained certainty of their spiritual invulnerability and their 'eternal form of existence'. This realisation is supported by the research into near-death experiences as described comprehensively, for example, by the Dutch cardiologist Pim van Lommel.[20]

---

[18] See Aaron Antonovsky, *Salutogenese. Zur Entmystifizierung von Gesundheit* [Salutogenesis. Demystification of health]. Tübingen: dgvt Verlag, 1997; Antonovsky, Aaron. 1983. *The Sense of Coherence: Development of a Research Instrument.* W.S. Schwartz Research Center for Behavioral Medicine, Tel Aviv University, Newsletter and Research Reports 1/1983.
[19] See Abraham Maslow, *Religions, Values and Peak-Experiences*. Columbus: Ohio State University Press, 1964.
[20] See P. van Lommel, R. van Wees, V. Meyers and I. Elfferich, *Near-*

People who have had a near death experience and who have, therefore, experienced themselves in their eternal non-physical existence lose their fear of death and return to their daily life as a changed person with inner calm and stability. They have gained spiritual immunity. It is appropriate also in this context to talk of immunity as it stands for integrity and invulnerability.

Interestingly, the human biography is divided into three distinctive segments: during the first period the body develops and reaches its final shape and size in the $20^{th}/21^{st}$ year. During this time children and adolescents generally only contract illnesses which stimulate the immune system, i.e. infections of the upper respiratory tract, sore throat, otitis media (inflammation of the middle ear, infections of the gastro-intestinal system (digestive tract) and similar conditions.

The better a person's immune system develops during that first period, the healthier they will be during their whole adult life. During the second period, approximately between 20 and 45, a different group of illnesses emerges even when a person is basically healthy. These are the so-called psychosomatic illnesses: stomach-ache, headache, sensation of stabbing in the heart, disturbed sleep patterns, lack of appetite, lack of energy, a propensity for aggression, depression and so on. A doctor might prescribe medications to treat these symptoms and they may help for a while. However, it is often disappointing for the patient that the doctor cannot find an actual physical cause. Rather, the root of the discomfort is psychological – often comprising difficulties in adapting emotionally to a change in familial or

Death Experience in Survivors of Cardiac Arrest: A prospective Study in the Netherlands. In: The Lancet 2001 358(9298):2039–45;
P. van Lommel, P, Endloses Bewusstsein: Neue medizinische Fakten zur Nahtoderfahrung [Infinite consciousness: New medical facts on near death experiences]. Düsseldorf: Patmos, 2009.

work-related circumstances. These can be met by…

- Putting an end to the intolerable situation by leaving or resigning.

- Getting used to taking medication for the relief of symptoms and accepting possible side effects.

- Working on the soul's immune system' and becoming immune to everyday slights and grievances through self-development.

Countless coaching and self-help books give advice on self-development. Many magazines, too, regularly contain new articles on this topic, as it is of such fundamental importance. *Geo kompakt* published a whole issue (number 64, Oct 2020) on this topic with the headline: 'The power of confidence. How positive thinking can strengthen our body and soul.' The main chapters address the question 'Can hope heal us?', followed by the topics: 'Slowing down – how to create good quality of life', 'Resilience – can we emerge stronger from the corona crisis?' and 'Self-care – how to avoid stress.'

During the last third of our biography, which lasts until the end of our life, people suffer mainly from chronic health conditions. Not many people are entirely spared the experience of some form of chronic ailment. We find that our bodies no longer 'recover completely' after an illness as they used to. Instead, we realise that our physical strength and integrity diminish irreversibly, and the question arises more or less consciously: what will happen when our body breaks down completely and we die? Here, the concept of spiritual immunity comes to the fore: Will I continue to be myself even when my body disintegrates? Materialistically orientated science has no answer to this question, and many people gain support and solace in religious philosophies and beliefs.

In order to develop a deeper understanding in this area one has to search further. But how? No science or experimental evidence has so far managed convincingly to bridge the chasm between belief and knowledge, spirit and matter, super-sensible and physical sense perception. Is it even possible to prove spiritual realities by means of sense-perceptible facts? Moreover, how much sense does it even make to demand evidence for the existence of spirit? Isn't the human spirit the innermost being of man, his very own sphere of invisible inner dialogue? What use would external proof be for this inner dialogue? Do we not rather need personal conviction without being swayed by authority and stifling evidence? What's more, we only become certain of our own identity once we have freely decided what kind of person we want to be. Is not the insurmountable chasm or the so-called threshold between the sensory and super-sensory worlds the best proof for the fact that evolution (or however we wish to call its creator) has granted human beings the capacity for freedom?

Animals show us in a wonderful way that nature can create perfect beings with a clear identity who are not plagued by self-doubt and torments of conscience. Why is man not endowed with this perfection? Why is man deficient from birth, having to supplement his imperfect instincts through active learning and to shape his identity through hard work? This difficult question is often addressed by great philosophers and artists. For example, the protagonist in Goethe's *Faust* remarks, 'The nights seem to penetrate deeper / Only inside bright light shines' as he loses his sight towards the end of his life. How can we find the bright light inside without having to lose our physical eyesight?

Is there such a thing as a secular spirituality which is available to everyone, independent of their philosophical outlook and religious affiliation? Is not thinking itself the basis of this secular spirituality?

Life experience teaches us that we cannot enjoy even the sunniest, brightest day when we think bleak and self-destructive thoughts. We experience the power which thoughts can exert over us. The same is true for our feelings. Their relative warmth or coldness lead us to constructive or destructive attitudes and actions, respectively. We also realise how much our thoughts about other people and the world are influenced by the ideas which we formed during our early upbringing and education. When we become aware of this we may want to pause and consider whether we want to remain at that level for the rest of our life. Is this really how I see myself as a human being? Or are there totally different possibilities of self-realisation – in the best sense of the word? And this is quite simply *the* ultimate question of conscience. Because my answer to this question will determine the quality of my inner guidance – will it be good or bad, or sensitive to my evolutionary potential? (More on this below.)

The answer to this question will also impact my sense of health. If I feel torn internally, if I reject or even hate myself, compare myself to others and put myself down, then I create inner harm and pain which in turn weaken my immune system. Immunity means being invulnerable and autonomous. The foundations for this are independent thought and judgement. It is always one's self-determination and self-actualisation which strengthen the immune system on the physical, mental/emotional and spiritual levels. Ultimately, what gives lasting strength for the soul is the experience and development of one's own personality, the 'I' as the spiritual core of the human being. In this regard, the self-development book by Rudolf Steiner, *'Knowledge of Higher Worlds'*[21], has helped me a lot – personally, and professionally in my work with patients.

---

21 Rudolf Steiner, *How to Know Higher Worlds: A modern path of initiation*. Collected Works (CW) no. 10. Various editions. Originally titled (in English): *Knowledge of the Higher Worlds and Its Attainment.*

Freedom and Dignity –
the psychosomatic signature
of the heart

Man is free insofar as he is able to follow himself at every moment of his life.
Rudolf Steiner

The so-called powerlessness of the individual is perhaps the most dangerous illusion which a person can ever have.
Joseph Weizenbaum

In the summer of 1984 Joseph Weizenbaum (1923-2008), professor of computer science at the Massachusetts Institute of Technology (MIT) in Cambridge, USA, and world-renowned specialist in computer technology, gave an interview with Bernhard Moosbrugger of Piper-Verlag (publishers). It was the famous year of George Orwell's novel '1984'. The obvious question was whether computers would enable complete control of society in the near future. Weizenbaum stated outright: 'I would not dream of saying that a police state, like Orwell described it, could not happen: we are already working towards it with every means at our disposal! And many who fear that Big Brother will soon be watching their every move and listening to their every telephone call, are nonetheless contributing to the development of devices which, when viewed in the current historic context, can only be seen as tools intended for policing.

But if this kind of state becomes a reality it will be much more a consequence of people no longer defending their freedom rather than the fault of the computer. For example, at the time of the Romanovs there already existed a secret police in Russia. This shows that a surveillance state can also be implemented without a computer. Stalin and Hitler also got by without a computer! So, when a totalitarian state comes into being, it is not primarily due to a device but rather because people do not sufficiently stand up for their values.' [22]

Interestingly, unlike the brain the heart is not an organ of control. Rather, it is a sensitive organ of perception for the needs of the organism. And yet it remains completely autonomous, much more so than the brain which can survive undamaged only for a few minutes without blood flow. And who controls the heart? No-one!

Already during my medical studies, I was excited to learn that the heart is autonomous, a 'free' organ as it were. The heart muscle is able to self-activate independently of the nerve supply, whose only function is modification. This impulse spreads to the entire myocardium and then relaxes again. The heartbeat is the result of an autonomous generation and conduction of this impulse. The heart is thus able to 'follow itself', as Rudolf Steiner states in his book *Philosophy of Freedom* about free human beings.[23] This feat is accomplished by the sinoatrial node (the 'pacemaker'), which is located in the right atrial wall, and its connected system of conduction fibres which reach into the ventricles. If the sinoatrial node fails to set the normal rhythm

---

[22] Joseph Weizenbaum, *Kurs auf den Eisberg: Die Verantwortung des Einzelnen und die Diktatur der Technik* [Heading for the Iceberg: The responsibility of the individual and the dictatorship of technology]. München und Zürich: Piper, 1987.

[23] Rudolf Steiner, *The Philosophy of Freedom*. CW 4. Various editions.

(60-80 beats per minute) due to illness, then the atrioventricular node (part of the cardiac conduction system located between the atria and ventricles) takes on this role with a slower rhythm of 40 beats per minute. Should this also fail then the endings of the cardiac conduction system, which are located in the ventricles, can keep the heart beating with approx. 20 beats per minute, creating the so-called idioventricular rhythm.[24]

What constitutes the dignity of the heart? What gives a person dignity? This comes definitely through autonomy with its associated sovereignty. It is also, of course, through the way in which someone expresses their autonomy towards other people, including within larger social contexts. If this expression is egoistical and self-centred then it is experienced as 'undignified'. But if the person succeeds in balancing the necessary self-care with the empathic bond and concern for the whole then they become a positive example for humanity. The physiological archetype for this can be seen in the position and role of the heart in the organism: it is the autonomous centre of the whole organism and faithfully accompanies a human being from day 21 until their death. It beats tirelessly day and night, and whoever is able to observe it by ultrasound scans will see how full of vigour it cheerfully beats away.

The opening and closing of the heart valves which separate the atria from the ventricles look like small ballerinas who gracefully open their arms and hands upwards and outwards and then close them again. When we use the phrase 'hand on heart' which invites someone to speak with total honesty these are not empty words. The heart can be seen as the organic correspondence or the instrument of the human 'I'. Not for nothing does Mephistopheles state the famous words in Goethe's Faust,

---

[24]   see Vaupel et.al., op.cit. p.213-14.

'Blood is a very special fluid'. The holy sacrament of the transubstantiation of bread and wine is centred around the blood and the body which it serves. It is not surprising therefore that the blood is the carrier of the immune system, i.e. the carrier of our biological identity, and that our mental and psychological states strongly influence the health of our blood and our immune system. How can we explain this reciprocal relationship?

The anthroposophic view of the human being offers a starting hypothesis, namely, that bodily principles metamorphose from physical to non-physical/spiritual orientation. But what is idea or thought realism? It is the philosophical current going back to Plato and to the debate struggling against nominalism in the Middle Ages, holding that ideas and concepts or thoughts were not insubstantial shadows, merely names or 'nouns' (as the nominalists expounded), but were realities in themselves.

In German idealism and early romanticism, this idea-realism was revived in the philosophical debates with Kant. Rudolf Steiner built on this in his book *Philosophy of Freedom*, making it practicable as the basis for anthroposophic knowledge of the human being and of the self.[25]

Steiner discovered that the principles which govern growth, differentiation, and development of the whole body both in embryonal configuration and after birth do not only work on the physical level. They are also spiritual forces and principles which, although not perceptible with the normal senses, are experienced by the growing human being as his emerging inner life in the form of thoughts, feelings and will impulses.

Steiner formulated this law he had discovered of the metamor-

---

[25]   See Peter Heusser's book, *Anthroposophy and Science*, Peter Lang publishers, 2016.

phosis of the body-configuring and body-related principles, which he calls members or 'principles' [26] of the human being, into non-physical soul-spiritual activity as follows:

'It is of the greatest importance to know that ordinary human powers of thought are refined powers of morphological configuration and growth. A spiritual principle reveals itself in the configuration and growth of the human organism, and as life progresses this principle emerges as the spiritual power of thought. And this power of thought is only one part of the power of human configuration and growth that is at work in the etheric. The other part remains faithful to the function it had at the beginning of human life. Human beings continue to develop when configuration and growth have reached an advanced stage, that is, to some degree a conclusion. It is because of this that the non-physical, spiritual-etheric, which is alive and actively at work in the organism, is able to become power of thought in later life. The power to change and be changed thus presents itself to imaginative perception in one aspect as being the etheric and spiritual, and in its other aspect as the soul content of thinking.' [27]

Steiner's description of the relationship between the etheric organisation (the principles which make life possible) and the activity of thought also applies respectively to the relationship between the astral organisation (the principles which govern sensation and emotions) and feeling, and to the relationship be-

---

[26] *Wesensglieder* in German, variously translated in Steiner's writings as members, principles, organisations or bodies of the human being, depending on publication and context.

[27] Rudolf Steiner, Ita Wegman. *Extending Practical Medicine. Fundamental Principles Based on the Science of the Spirit.* CW 27. London: Rudolf Steiner Press, 2020. Translated by Anne Meuss.

tween the 'I' organisation (the principles which allow for the experience of the innermost self in the body) and the will. This is the basis of the psychosomatic concept in anthroposophic understanding of the human being. The soul faculties of thinking, feeling and will, which each person has responsibility for guiding, are in fact principles which have become freed from nature's laws and body-related activity. Nature's wisdom (the laws of physical nature) ceases to apply in human beings. The human being owes his deficient nature and his inadequate instincts to the fact that these wisdom-filled laws leave the body in the course of growth and development and are transformed into the abilities to think, feel and willing. The influences of these three complex principles which facilitate life, ensoulment and self-awareness, can be observed particularly well during the embryonal development.

In the first week only that principle is active which enables the building up of matter, i.e. the physical organisation. This leads to an increase of substance without any overall growth in size as part of the process of division, which is characteristic for the first embryonic week (see Figure 5).

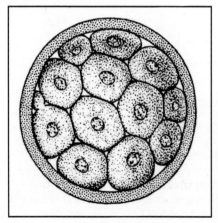

Figure 5: After fertilisation cell divisions begin to occur, the so-called cleavage, which lead to the multiplication of cells without any increase in size of the fertilised egg. Cell growth only begins once the egg is implanted in the mother's uterus.

During the second week differentiation begins on the one hand of the embryonic tissue into sheaths (umbilical vesicle or yolk sac, allantois, connecting stalk and chorion) and on the other hand of the developing embryo which is located inside the sheaths. We can see in this typical aspects of life governing principles: in centre and periphery, the living organism within its milieu.

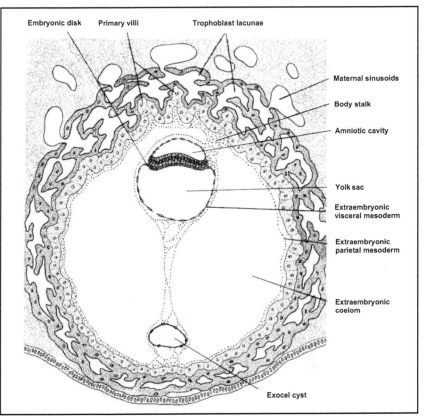

Figure 6 shows the embryo at the end of the second week after successful implantation. It only consists of two cell layers: the outer cell layer (ectoderm) adjacent to the amniotic sac (amnion); and the inner cell layer (endoderm) adjoining the yolk sac. So, the surrounding structures are created first, i.e. the membranes which envelop the embryo: the trophoblast which later forms the placenta; the amnion, the yolk sac and the connecting stalk which will fuse to form the umbilical cord.

Only in week three do the embryonic cells begin to differentiate and with this the development of the mesoderm, from which the heart and blood formation arise. The process of growth is now joined by the processes of differentiation and configuration of cell structures and organ systems.

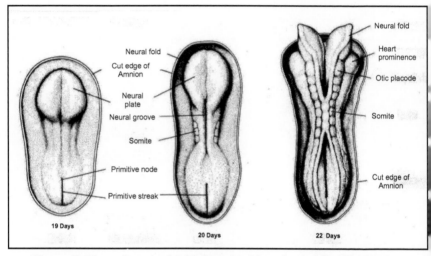

Figure 7: The embryo in the third week without its sheaths. The head-trunk area and the metabolic system begin to form. Already at the end of week three the heart begins to beat (which is not shown in this illustration).

In week four the foetal outline becomes visible for the first time due to the workings of a unifying principle which brings all the parts together and integrates them into a whole. In the further course of development, these principles which configure the complex human constitution work in ever greater harmony.

When we examine the dynamics of our own thinking, feeling and will, we can sense the same signature at work: thoughts in the form of mental pictures, conceptions, ideas and ideals have an incredibly extensive creative potential which can be used in constructive or destructive ways. The so-called thought life is

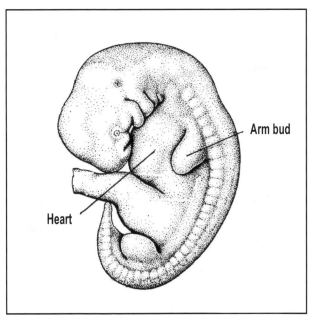

Figure 8: At the end of week four the embryo appears as an integral shape for the first time – inclusive of the small buds that will grow into arms and legs. The configuration of the evolving human form is clearly orchestrated by a holistically coordinating system of forces.

creative, formative and productive. On the other hand feelings we experience as forces not in picture form but rather of a more musical nature and differentiated in themselves. And the will-life is characterised by the ability to focus exclusively on an intended action. Taking this further, a person experiences their 'I' in self-directed actions, self-development and a self-regulation which directs the whole 'human system'. As a rule, the 'self' becomes mentally aware only in the third year, when it begins to wonder who it really is who has been crawling, has become upright and has spoken – namely the 'I', the child's individuality.

Steiner used the term incarnation for the process of connecting and identifying with our own physical form (called embodiment in modern research). Incarnation, though, opens the prospect of a purely spiritual pre-birth existence consisting of the forces which configure the physical, etheric, soul and 'I'-endowed being. As growth and biographical ageing advance from embryonal development, childhood and youth to older age these forces free themselves again from their physical tasks and become available for the soul-spiritual experiences of thinking, feeling and will. In this inner experiential space we can reflect on our existence before birth and after death and become aware of our eternal being, i.e. our spiritual origin. Looked at in this way, human life becomes a soul-spiritual embryonal development up to the point of death, which is then a complete 'excarnating birth' out of the physical body which has become useless.

Where does the transition occur from the incarnating to the excarnating work of the bodily principles? There really is only one place where this can happen. It must be a place, or rather an organ, where life activity can be brought to a standstill for brief periods during which the physically focussed, life enabling activities of the bodily principles can withdraw and transform into the spiritual processes. This place is the heart. The blood circulation, which is in constant motion throughout the organism, comes to a standstill for a fraction of a second in the heart (as noted on page 30). In this moment, the amount of blood which flows into the heart makes a U-turn of 180degrees – a reversal of direction from the venous inflow to the arterial outflow. This means that every unit of flow must go through a zero point, which can be likened to a small moment of death.[28]

---

[28] See Michaela Glöckler, *Was kann die Pädagogik zur Prävention von Herz-Kreislauf-Erkrankungen leisten?* [What can pedagogy contribute to the prevention of cardiovascular diseases?], in *Das menschliche Herz. Kardiologie in der anthroposophischen Medizin* [The Human Heart. Cardiology in anthroposophic medicine] edited by Christoph Rubens and Peter Selg, Arlesheim: Verlag des Ita Wegman Instituts, 2014; Armin Husemann,

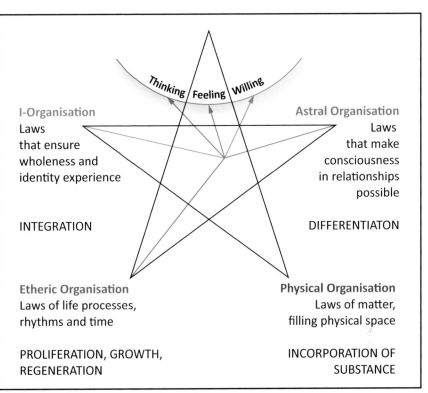

Figure 9: Schematic diagram of the psychosomatic paradigm showing the four bodily principles working in the body, and their non-physical functions of thinking, feeling, will ('Quinta Essentia')

This brief 'moment of death' allows the individual bodily principles to detach from the physical constitution and to integrate into the 'Quinta Essentia'. This fifth being is seen by all cultures as spiritual in nature - in contrast to the four elements earth, water, air, fire. The concept of the 'Quinta Essentia' was already known to Aristotle, who regarded the four elements not as substances but as principles - in the sense of what is described as 'aggregate states' in physics. The phrase 'thinking with the heart' is surely connected to this.

Die Blutbewegung und das Herz [The movement of blood and the heart], Stuttgart: Freies Geistesleben, 2019.

We have a distinct feeling for how the soul forces become conscious in the head through perceptual and reflective thought activity, but that they do not arise there. For a thought to become heartfelt, I must get excited by it, emotionally connect with it, and then also realise it. The thoughts, feelings and will impulses flow imperceptibly from the heart to the head and surround us in the form of the so-called soul-spiritual aura. We become conscious of some of those thoughts, feelings and intentions and not of others, depending on our manifold life experiences. If we direct the conscious thoughts, feelings and intentions back to the heart, we acquire warm human radiance of freedom and dignity for our actions and aspirations.

Autonomy and conscience

Yet keep your spirit free!
Never lose yourself!
No heaven will make
Amends for this loss.
Do not forget yourself in the feeling of wretchedness.
Friedrich Hölderlin

As long as I only think about something I remain completely free because I can discard the thought at any time. Before I reject a thought, though, I think it completely through and relate it to what I already know through my life experience. I examine whether the thought makes sense and feels true, and whether it can expand and enrich my understanding of the world.

Only then do I decide whether to follow this thought or not. This method of internal scrutiny by means of one's own thinking and powers of observation has an advantage over scientific research: no large sums of money are needed to prepare, plan and conduct a study, neither does one need to wait for results. Rather, if one resonates with a good thought one can act on it directly and observe whether it works or not. Life itself will reveal whether the thought is helpful and congruent. Independent thinking positions us in real life rather than in a laboratory. This way of thinking and discerning is called common sense. Thinking seems all the healthier the truer it is to reality and life. This is why Rudolf Steiner appealed again and again to people's common sense when he talked about his spiritual insights and research findings (Anthroposophy). He said, not everyone would have the ability to verify his research findings through their own spiritual perception. However, anyone could assess in their own life whether spiritual insights made sense, and whether they promoted or impeded one's understanding of self and the world.

> *Those who apply it correctly will find that the knowledge of spiritual science proves itself in life by making life strong and healthy. They will see it is true because it is valid in life and practice, and in this they will find a proof stronger than all the logical, so-called scientific arguments can afford. Spiritual truths are best recognised by their fruits and not by what is called a proof, no matter how scientific.* [29]

The same is true for the messages from the voice of conscience. Often there are two voices which speak up and they sometimes conflict with each other. One voice affirms and justifies what we have done – this is the so-called clear conscience. The other voice raises doubt and guilt and chips away at our soul, influencing us with negative feelings. Both types of intuition should be examined before we 'believe' them or even rashly follow them, especially since common experience shows that the male constitution tends toward a clear conscience, whereas women are more likely to find fault with themselves and take the blame. If a male-female-couple share an experience, for example, which resonates in different ways in their souls (as described above) it is extremely helpful to discuss it and to assess the situation consciously in order to approach the truth. But what is the truth? Is not the 'right' thing that which serves life? A habitually good conscience tempts us to stagnate in our evolution and to be-

[29]   Rudolf Steiner, *The Education of the Child*, CW34, Anthroposophic Press 1996, p.36.

come self-satisfied – whatever our experiences are. Sooner or later this leads to problems in social relationships. The permanently bad conscience also leads to a developmental dead end – to low moods, self-doubt and depression. If one is unaware of this, one easily becomes dependent on friends and acquaintances who give advice and try to help, or on therapeutic or spiritual authorities who can give professional support.

So how can we do justice to life and thereby foster autonomy, health and truthfulness? We can do it by preserving our good judgement, by hearing all our inner voices of conscience – not only the 'automatic' ones - and also carefully evaluating them as to their validity. Is there also a voice which only speaks when we in all honesty ask a direct question? For example, 'what can I learn from this situation? What could I do better if I found myself in a similar situation in the future? Allow myself to be more open? Listen better, say 'no' more firmly, be more decisive?' If I keep asking myself these kinds of questions I will receive guidance, especially if I take them into my sleep at night when wrestling with a difficult situation. Guidance might not necessarily come the next morning but rather sometime during the day when I do not expect it. This voice is different from the other two voices in that it prompts us and yet leaves us completely free.

Interestingly, in his Christological lectures Rudolf Steiner kept emphasising how valuable and appropriate it is that there is no real scientific proof (in the sense of natural science) that Christ-Jesus lived on earth, let alone that he was resurrected from death on the cross.

Especially in reference to the Christ-Event it must be understood in our time that one can only come to the Christ in a spiritual way. He will never truly be found by external methods. We may be told that Christ exists, but to find Him really is only possible by spiritual means. It is important to consider that concerning the Christ-Event, all who do not admit to spiritual insight must live with a misunderstanding about it.[30]

If we realise, however, that our voice of conscience already is a possibility for conveying spiritual insight, we can experience Christ's closeness, the fact that he is with us 'all the days until the completion of earthly time' (Matthew 28:20). [31]

When Christ inspires our conscience in situations of remorse, then it sounds healing and encouraging. It gives us the confidence that learning and new developmental steps are possible and that they will serve ourselves and others. In situations when we feel self-righteous, though, it will inspire us to see ourselves in the larger context and develop the readiness to grow through the experience.

The early medieval monk and scholar Johannes Scotus Eriugena (9th century) composed a literary dialogue called Periphyseon / De divisione naturae - or 'about the division of nature'. Here is a summary of some of his questions and answers relevant in this context:

- What do humans have in common with minerals? Answer: the physical body.

- What do humans have in common with plants?

[30]   Rudolf Steiner, The Forming of Destiny After Death, CW157a, 1989, Garber Communications, Blauvelt, NY; alternate translation in Rudolf Steiner, *Spiritual Life Now and After Death: Forming Our Destiny in the Physical and Spiritual Worlds*, CW157a, SteinerBooks, 2013.
[31]   Biblical quotes from the Jon Madsen translation, *The New Testament*, Floris books, 2017.

Answer: life.

- What do humans have in common with animals?
  Answer: the soul.

- What do humans have in common with angels?
  Answer: thinking.

- What does man have in common with no one else, but
  only himself? Independent judgment.

In a certain sense we stand between the material and the super-sensible/non-material worlds when we consult with ourselves and with our conscience; in other words, we stand between the world of the senses and the world of the spirit, which is only accessible through thinking. In this place, we are totally on our own, but we are also open to what can inspire us from the spiritual super-sensible world. Loneliness and connectedness do not contradict each other - neither in the sense world nor in the spiritual world. We need both, so we can recognise ourselves as autonomous beings, and integrate ourselves consciously and meaningfully into the totality of our environment.

The Heart as wellspring of longing and conscience

I feel a long and unresolved desire
For that serene and solemn land of ghosts:
It quivers now, like an Aeolian lyre,
My stuttering verse, with its uncertain notes,
A shudder takes me: tear on tear, entire,
The firm heart feels weakened and remote:
What I possess seems far away from me,
And what is gone becomes reality.
            Johann Wolfgang von Goethe, Faust I, Dedication [32]

Goethe's drama begins and ends in heaven, i.e. in the spiritual world where there are beings who promote human evolution, but also those who endeavour to thwart man's evolution and who aim to lead him astray. It does not take much to realise that the development towards freedom is only possible in the way expressed in the Gospel of John: 'You will recognise the truth, and the truth will lead you to freedom' (John 8:32). Goethe devoted his 'Faust' to this quest for truth, working on it right up into his last year of life. At the beginning of the play, Faust has thoughts of suicide. At the threshold to the spirit realms he is distracted from this by the sound of Easter bells and beautiful memories of childhood. He then intentionally links his fate

---

[32]   A.S. Kline translation - source for this and the following Goethe quote from: https://www.poetryintranslation.com/

with Mephistopheles – the 'spirit that always denies', and 'always intends evil but always creates good' – and accompanies him throughout his life. In the end, his wanderings and experiences lead him to the vision of the free human being (Part II, Act V, Scene VI):

Yes, I've surrendered to this thought's insistence,
The last word Wisdom ever has to say:
He only earns his Freedom and Existence,
Who's forced to win them freshly every day. ...
I wish to gaze again on such a land,
Free earth: where a free race, in freedom, stands.
Then, to the Moment I'd dare say:
'Stay a while! You are so lovely!'
Through aeons, then, never to fade away
This path of mine through all that's earthly.

Although we use our head to think about the voice of conscience, it is the heart which can discern the different nuances of our conscience, and even react by constricting or feeling light and at ease. The heart responds immediately to our feelings; indeed, it is the centre of our feeling life. And this includes longings – the longing for health, for the fulfilment of our desires and hopes, and the achievement of our self-determined goals. There is the longing for identity and security, for a new innocence, purity, love, trust, hope, confidence and truth – ultimately, a longing for transformation and wholeness. Our heart also holds the longing for new beginnings, for leaving the past behind and to change, for meeting new challenges, for looking at our past with fresh eyes and to come to terms with it. Thus, the heart is an organ which ceaselessly opens itself up and closes in on itself. The same rhythm is needed by our feeling life when we open ourselves to the problems of this world, but then,

63

too, clearly consider our inner capacities - examining whether or not they enable us to contribute to a solution. The ability of our heart to open itself can be likened to our ability to open ourselves for the inspirations whispered by the voice of conscience – the 'coming home' to the prevailing state of emotions and the desires, hopes and longings connected with them.

The romantic poet Friedrich von Hardenberg, known as Novalis (1772-1801), extends our view of human conscience in the unfinished second part of his novel 'Heinrich von Ofterdingen'. Heinrich meets a physician called Sylvester. To begin with they talk about nature and the forces of the elements which can create violent weather conditions, making Earth a living hell; and yet they can also produce crystal clear skies with delicate white clouds. Sylvester compares this to the nature of the human voice of conscience. A conversation ensues about the true nature of man's conscience which Sylvester calls the heavenly conscience or the 'higher nature of man'.

He says, 'These are echoes of a primitive inhuman nature, but also summoning voices of a higher nature, of heavenly conscience in us. The mortal roars in its deeps; the immortal begins to shine brighter and comes to know itself.'

'When,' asked Henry, 'will the need for all fear, all pain, all want and all evil be removed from the universe?'

'When there is only one power – the power of conscience. – When nature has become modest and moral. There is only one cause of evil – common weakness. And this weakness is nothing but poor ethical receptivity, a lack of charm in freedom.'

'Do please make the nature of conscience comprehensible to me.'

'If I could do that, I would be God, for conscience arises in the very act of understanding it...' '...conscience appears in every serious completion, in every embodied truth. Every inclination and skill which reflection turns into a world-image becomes a phenomenon, a transmutation of conscience. Indeed, all development leads to what can only be called freedom, regardless of the fact that thereby not simply a mere concept but the creative basis of all existence is to be designated. This freedom is mastery. The master exercises unfettered power in a purposeful, definite, and deliberate manner. The objects of his art are his and subject to his pleasure, and they do not shackle or cramp him. And precisely this all-embracing freedom, mastery, or sovereignty is the essence, the drive of conscience. In him is revealed the holy peculiarity, the immediate creativity of personality, and every act of the master is at the same time a proclamation of the lofty, simple, uncomplicated world – God's word...'

'Conscience is man's most peculiar essence in full transfiguration, the divine primal man. It is not just this or that; its throne is not set on general maxims, nor does it consist of single virtues. There is only one virtue: the pure earnest will which at the moment of decision resolves and chooses without mediation. In living, peculiar indivisibility it inhabits and animates the delicate symbol of the human body and is able to put all the spiritual members into the truest activity.' [33]

Thereafter, their conversation returns to the art of poetry which Heinrich now recognises as an expression of the voice of conscience.

This inspired description of human conscience gives voice to <u>something which</u> can only really be understood once it has

[33] Novalis, *Heinrich von Ofterdingen* [Henry of Ofterdingen], Trans. Prof. Palmer Hilty, New York: Frederick Ungar Publishing, 1964, pp 164-6.

been experienced. Novalis' account offers us four ways towards comprehending the meaning of conscience:

- the innate mediator of each human being, the representative of God on Earth;

- the essence of freedom;

- man's very own being in full transfiguration, the divine primal man;

- a purely spiritual endeavour – the receiving of inspiration in full conscious awareness.

Novalis has thus characterised the issue which sparked the conversation between Heinrich and Sylvester. It is a question of self-knowledge, of the human 'I' as the innermost creative essence of human nature. We could also say that Novalis portrays that aspect of the voice of conscience which has been given many different names in literature and in religious writings: higher self, better or true self, the divine in man. St. Paul expressed it as 'Not I but Christ in me', or the so-called second birth through the formative powers of water and the breath of spirit (John 3:5).

Autonomy, secular spirituality and immunity

I ponder my heart
It quickens me
It warms me
I deeply trust
In the immortal self
Which weaves in me
Which carries me.
Rudolf Steiner

What is secular spirituality? Although Steiner never used this term, the spirituality studied in anthroposophic spiritual science is nonetheless secular because it bases itself on thinking as the bridge between the sensory world and the spirit world, just as thinking can create tangible images of sense impressions gathered by the sensory organs. Thinking, however, can completely detach itself from any sensory perception and be realised as a purely spiritual, conceptual-mathematical activity without any images at all. For example, any type of circle can be defined as the locus of points equidistant from the centre. However, we cannot form a mental image of the purely conceptual circle because as soon as we try to do so we leave the purely conceptual thinking behind and enter the realm of the sensorily imaginable.

Neither is ideational thinking connected to sense perceptions.

Instead, it is about judgements, 'good or bad ideas'- irrespective of their feasibility. And then there is the fourth category of ordinary thinking: idealistic thinking. Anyone who cherishes an ideal, for example the ideal of truth or honesty, knows very well that this goes beyond ordinary everyday thinking. The least interesting thing about the ideal of truth is the conceptual aspect of it. Whether I imagine an honest deed, whether I try to form a concept of truthfulness, or whether I have the great notion that from today onward I want to be honest and lie as little as possible does not really matter as far as the ideal itself is concerned. Honesty only becomes an ideal once I actually bring it to life, i.e. once the thought has become an impulse to act – we could even say once it has become part of my character and my identity.

Thus this simple reflection on the different types of thinking shows how spiritual (i.e. non-sensory, non-material) competency can build a bridge between what is given in the sense world, our mental pictures, and what is essentially spiritual. The extraordinary achievement of Anthroposophy is that it expresses spiritual realities in comprehensible thought forms and teaches us to observe the phenomena of the sense-perceptible world in such a way that they reveal more to us than we can see with our eyes and grasp with our hands.

Heart and Sun

In *The Sun as the Heart of the World* (1966) [34] Walther Bühler endeavoured to compare the sun with its great significance for all life on Earth to the human heart. Drawing on science, astronomy and spiritual science / anthroposophy, Bühler in an engaging way deepens not only our knowledge of the role of the sun in the universe but also our understanding of the essence and significance of the heart. Life on earth depends on the light of the sun which enables the plant world to produce chlorophyll and, therefore, energy. Human beings also depend in lots of ways on the direct exposure to sunlight. An obvious example is the production of vitamin D in our skin during exposure to sunlight. Research in recent decades has found that this 'sun vitamin' directly stimulates the innate and the adaptive immune systems. This explains why vitamin D is recommended in the treatment of many diseases – notably cancer, diabetes and autoimmune disorders[35], but also as part of the supportive treatment

---

[34]   Walther Bühler, *Die Sonne als Weltenherz*, Stuttgart: Verlag Freies Geistesleben, 1966. Not yet translated.

[35]   See Hector F. DeLuca, 'Overview of general physiologic features and functions of vitamin D', *The American Journal of Clinical Nutrition*, 80:6 (2004), pp. 1689-96; Michael F. Holick, 'Vitamin D: importance in the prevention of cancers, type 1 diabetes, heart disease, and osteoporosis', *The American Journal of Clinical Nutrition*, 79:3 (2004), pp. 362-371; E. Hyppönen, E. Läärä, A. Reunanen, M.R. Järvelin, S.M. Virtanen, 'Intake of vitamin D and risk of type 1 diabetes: a birth-cohort study', *Lancet*, 358:9292 (2001), pp. 1500-1503, (November 3, 2001); C.S. Zipitis, A.K. Akobeng, 'Vitamin D supplementation in early childhood and risk of type 1 diabetes: a systematic review and meta-analysis', Archives of Disease in Childhood, 2008, 93:6 (2008), pp. 512-517.

of Covid-19 patients.[36] Elderly people[37] as well as children are often deficient in Vitamin D and benefit from supplementation.

What the sun is for the evolution of the earth and its natural kingdoms, the cardiovascular system is for the human organism. Just as the sun is the central source of light and warmth for all life forms on earth, so the heart is the centre of the blood circulation which keeps all organs alive down to the smallest cells. There is a remarkable book aptly titled The Sun is to Blame, in which is described the importance of the sun for the entire evolution.[38] In this context we are reminded of Johannes Kepler's (1571-1630) fascination with the 'harmony of the spheres', including the rhythmic order of the sun, moon and earth, which he studied and wrote about. His observations led to his three well-known laws of planetary motion. Steiner repeatedly emphasised that the Earth-Sun relationship corresponds to the human biorhythms, especially in the rate of breathing. When calculated over a 24 hour period, the average rate of 18 breaths

---

[36]   See Mette M. Berger, Heike Bischoff-Ferrari, Isabelle Herter-Aeberli, Michael Zimmermann, Jörg Spieldenner, Manfred Eggersdorfer (An expert panel working with the Schweizerische Gesellschaft für Ernährung [Swiss Society for Nutrition] (SGE), 'Ausgewogene Ernährung und gezielte Nahrungsergänzung Effiziente Unterstützung bei der Bekämpfung der COVID-19-Pandemie' [Balanced diet and targeted nutritional supplements as effective support in combating the COVID-19 pandemic], *Schweizer Zeitschrift für Ernährungsmedizin* [Swiss Journal for Nutritional Medicine], 4 (2020), pp 19-21; White paper: *Nutritional status in supporting a well-functioning immune system for optimal health with a recommendation for Switzerland*, August 2020, https://tinyurl.com/3jyrp4e7; P. C. Calder et al, 'Optimal Nutritional Status for a Well-Functioning Immune System Is an Important Factor to Protect against Viral Infections', in *Nutrients* 2020, 12, 1181; doi:10.3390/nu12041181 (available at https://www.mdpi.com/2072-6643/12/4/1181)

[37]   See www.alterundmobilitaet.usz.ch/fachwissen/seiten/vitamin-d.aspx

[38]   Felix Sigel, *Schuld ist die Sonne: Das Fachbuch zu einer vergessenen Wissenschaft* [The sun is to blame: The textbook on a forgotten science]. New Trinity Media, 2013. Reprint of original edition, Moskau/Leipzig, 1975.

per minute leads to the famous platonic number 25,920. This equals the number of years, in the 'precession of the equinox', whereby the position of the Sun at the spring equinox against the background stars of the zodiac processes through the entire zodiac (a rate of 1 degree every 72 years, 360 degrees in 25,920 years) – known as the 'Platonic year'. Similarly, a time span of 18 years is needed for the earth's axis to complete its nutation and is related to these rhythms.[39]

The 17th century English physician, William Harvey, known for his discoveries on the circulation of blood, made further observations which are likely seen as inconsequential philosophical reflections by modern anatomists but could, on the other hand, be seen as central for a deeper understanding of the heart. In his book, On the Movement of the Heart and Blood in Animals (De motu cordis et sanquinis in animalibus, 1628), in the midst of describing for the first time the anatomical features and functions of the circulatory system, he pauses for reflection, comparing the heart with the sun, the heart as 'the primal source of life' and the sun as 'the heart of the world'.

'It is possible to call this movement a circulation in the same sense that Aristotle compared the weather and rain with a circular movement in the upper regions. For the moist earth warmed by the sun develops vapours; the rising vapours again densified to rain and fall downward again, moistening the earth. Here we have the circulation of the sun. In this and in similar manner through the movement of the sun, through its approach and retreat thunderstorms and other heavenly phenomena are abroad

---

[39]   Steiner describes how the Platonic year can be considered a great 'Day of the Heavens', with the nutational period part of a macrocosmic breath within that Day. 'This takes place just as many times in the macrocosmic year as the 18 breaths during the microcosmic day of 24 hours.' (in: *Man Hieroglyph of the Universe*, CW201, p54)

about. So also could possibly happen in the body that all parts are nourished, warmed and vitalised by way of a warmed, perfect common vapour like, spiritual and (if I may so express myself) nourishing blood, whereas the blood in the various parts of the body is cooled down, densified, and weakened and therefore returns to its origin, to the heart, it's source, to the altar of the body (lar = protective spirit of a house; hearth) in order to regain its perfection. There, through the naturally powerful fiery warmth, this treasure of life (vitae thesauro), liquified anew, is impregnated with spirit and with balsam, as it were, and from here it is again distributed: and all that is dependent upon the beating movement of the heart. Thus is the heart the primal source of life and the sun of the small world (principium vitae et sol microcosmi), just as the sun in the same relationship deserves to be named the heart of the world. By virtue of this force and its beat the blood is moved, brought to perfection, nourished, and preserved from decay and disintegration. By nourishing, warming and vitalising, the heart in turn provides services to the entire body – this household god, the basis of life, the originator of all being. The heart is the root of the lives of living beings, the lord of them all, the sun of the small world upon which depends all life and from which radiates all freshness and all force.' [40]

Yet no matter how many analogies we use to describe the sun as the giver of life, the heart of our world, and the centre of the macrocosm to which we belong – they only ever give an external perspective. Is there also an internal perspective of the sun? That place where all the wisdom is gathered which manifests in the solar activities and their effects on the evolution on earth?

[40]   This translation of Harvey (original in Latin) from *The Anthroposophical Approach to Medicine* by F. Husemann and O. Wolf, Vol II, Anthroposophic Press, Spring Valley, NY, 1987. Translated (from the German) by Lisa Davisson.

Is there such a thing as a solar consciousness where all the wise thoughts and principles converge? Moreover, is there a Sun Spirit? Is there a Sun Soul which, in an all-encompassing yet very personal way, feels for the well-being of all those creatures who rely on it? Can we only have an outer material relationship to the sun, or can we also have a spiritual inner relationship with this powerful life centre of our evolution?

The pre-Christian mysteries venerated the sun and other planetary deities. What is the origin of this reverence? Who is Ahura Mazdao in the old Persian religion? Is it conceivable that the sun spirit so completely freed itself from all power that it could unite with a human body, with Jesus of Nazareth, through the baptism in the Jordan and then spend three years on earth amongst human beings, ending his life in the sacrificial deed on Golgotha? Is it possible that his risen spirit might walk with all human beings as a personal, spiritual companion – providing inner light and strength, and a loving, encouraging inner voice which gives hope? It has always deeply touched me that the German word 'Ich' ('I') is made up of the initials I.Ch., i.e. Jesus Christus. Just as everyone uses the word 'Ich' when they refer to themselves and describe their most personal aspects, they still share this name 'Ich' or 'I' with all other people.

What might emerge if we gazed at the sky, the sun and the stars with such contemplations and feelings - rather than simply looking at the external appearances and formulating scientific theories? It surely would change us and our relationship to our world. And it would explain why Novalis speaks of a 'heavenly conscience' which inspires not only each individual human being but also inspired the evangelists and great founders of religions. It is not human beings who are God's representatives on earth but the heavenly conscience which speaks to us through the heart. Thinking, when seen as a secular spirituality, encompasses the whole 'thinkable' world. It is not related to any particular religious orientation, and yet we depend on it for everything we know about God and the world.

Conclusion

Just as a physician is ultimately accountable only to his own conscience – by virtue of the Hippocratic oath – so can we also practise this ourselves on a free and voluntary basis. This decision alone, in the last instance to answer to our own true self, to the innermost voice of our conscience instead of to the state, church or science, energises our independent thinking, gives courage and strengthens the heart, and thus our immune system. Of course we take into account the regulations, anxieties and fears connected with the Corona Pandemic; however, we are also secure in the inner knowledge – in terms of the five gateways to illness and health – that decisions about life and death do not depend on regulations made by the authorities. Rather, they are deeply connected to our own destiny, and our development does not stop when we die. This kind of attitude and inner certainty allows us to distinguish between regulations which truly serve life and those which are absurd, an end unto themselves, out of touch with life and, what is more, are undermining the right to freedom in democratic societies. To regard safety higher than freedom means to conform to a materialistic logic and to serve the concentration of power. When we come to terms with the fact that the only sure thing in life is death, we become free to truly live and appreciate every precious moment of our life. As Novalis put it:

'The heart is the key to the world and to life. Man lives in this vulnerable condition so he can love and commit to others. Our imperfection allows us to be touched by others, and this external influence is the whole point. When we are ill only others should and can help us. Seen from this perspective Christ is indeed the key to the world.' [41]

If we want to avoid a 'health dictatorship', the individual must become more aware of the foundations of individual and social health, and of what a healthcare system worthy of the name would look like. The central question, though, is, 'Who is responsible for my health and for the kind of lifestyle I lead? Which risks am I willing and able to take, and where does the responsibility of the state lie?'

The Corona pandemic clearly shows that arrangements must be found which enable people to have a say in the consultations and decisions about their health. Already 100 years ago Rudolf Steiner talked about the need for democratising the health service. He spoke of the informed patient who meets the physician eye to eye and shares the responsibility for his own health. We need an education for the freedom of the individual, and a suitable legal-political framework supporting this. Otherwise one can foresee that people will become progressively dependent on prevailing authoritative views and political-economic power structures.

In an interview with Spiegel (German news magazine, transl.) on 2nd Dec 2020 to the question of how governments could counteract the problem of loneliness, the well-known economist and critic of capitalism, Noreena Hertz, said in reply: [42] :

'They should regulate social media more closely, especially

---

[41] Novalis, *Treplitzer Fragmente, Nr. 62* [Treplitz Fragments].
[42] Noreena Hertz, *The Lonely Century: Coming Together in a World that's Pulling Apart*, London: Sceptre, 2020.

when it comes to children. Social media are the tobacco industry of the 21st century. Outlaw the networks which lead children under 16 into addiction.'

Spiegel: 'That sounds fundamentalist.'

Hertz: 'Do you know that many of the people who built Silicon Valley keep their children away from smart phones and the internet for as long as possible? They do not give their children any iPads and they send them to Waldorf schools. Why? Because they know that social media are addictive – they know the algorithms. The more these people know about social media the less they want their children to use them.'

When people follow their conscience and have the courage to speak the truth, even when it is unpopular, without the fear of stigmatisation or exclusion, not only is the immune system strengthened but also people's trust in the future.

List of Illustrations

Figures 1a and 1b from www.euromomo.eu/graphs-and-maps/

Figures 2 and 3 from Autonomie der Blutbewegung: Ein neuer Blick auf Herz und Kreislauf [Autonomous movement of the blood: a new perspective on the heart and circulation], by Branko Furst, MD, Berlin: Salumed Verlag, 2020. Reprinted by kind permission of the publishers and author.

Figure 4 by A. Rad and M. Häggström. Creative Commons CC-BY-SA 3.0 license, via Wikimedia Commons.

Figures 5-8 from Wolfgang Schad, Die Vorgeburtlichkeit des Menschen [Human prenatal development], Stuttgart: Urachhaus, 1983.

Figure 9 from Michaela Glöckler, Education for the Future, Stroud: InterActions, 2020, p. 66.

Original German
for verses in the text

Spirit triumphant
Flame through the weakness
Of faint-hearted souls...

> *Sieghafter Geist*
> *Durchflamme die Ohnmacht*
> *Zaghafter Seelen.*
> *Verbrenne die Ichsucht,*
> *Entzuende das Mitleid,*
> *Dass Selbstlosigkeit,*
> *Der Lebensstrom der Menschheit,*
> *Wallt als Quelle*
> *Der geistigen Wiedergeburt.*
>
> Rudolf Steiner

keep your spirit free!
Never lose yourself!...

> *Doch erhalte den Geist dir frei!*
> *Verliere nie dich selbst!*
> *Für diesen Verlust entschädiget*
> *kein Himmel dich.*
> *Vergiß dich nicht*
> *im Gefühle der Dürftigkeit!*
>
> Friedrich Hölderlin

I ponder my heart
It quickens me
It warms me
I deeply trust
In the immortal self
Which weaves in me
Which carries me.

Ich denke an mein Herz
Es belebet mich
Es erwärmet mich
Ich vertraue fest
Auf das ewige Selbst
Das in mir wirket
Das mich trägt.

Rudolf Steiner

Appendix[1]

For a necessary rethinking of Corona politics and a greater understanding of the diversity of opinions in crises.

By Michaela Glöckler MD and Andreas Neider

The Corona Pandemic is not only an extremely complex event in terms of health, but it has also come at a time of great environmental, social and geopolitical change, and it is in itself a part of these changes. According to UNICEF, the pandemic will add another 130 million people to the 700 million who suffer from hunger worldwide, in addition to the problems we all face in the form of climate, hunger and poverty crises - accompanied by armed conflicts, refugee misery and hardship. These changes and hardships require a rethinking on both a large and small scale.

The Pandemic and the way it has been managed have confronted most of the world's population with the fact that much of what was taken for granted until recently has suddenly ceased to exist: the daily drive or walk to work, to kindergarten and school, the personal freedom of movement, shopping, participation in cultural events, weddings, funerals, family celebrations, leisure activities, and much more.

The screen has become the central meeting and communication place. However, the accelerated digitization of all areas of life is not only experienced as a blessing. Children and young people need first and foremost real-world experiences and contacts for their healthy development.

[1]   Amended from the original essay published in German at Easter 2021. Figures within the text have been amended to reflect status for August 2021. The translation for this Appendix text is by Astrid Schmitt-Stegmann.

In addition, there is concern whether the consistent tracking of infection chains and vaccination proofs, as well as other control and monitoring instruments that are deemed necessary, will lead to a future in which we have to reckon that they will be used again at any time when national emergencies such as the threat of terrorism or pandemics occur. How must democracy be developed further, so that fear of violence, of disease and death does not become the enemy of freedom and individual rights?

Many people are asking themselves, what kind of future is in store for us? What kind of citizen participation is needed to keep democracy viable in the face of this changed overall situation? How can civil society be concretely involved in the process of a necessary rethinking - also in Corona politics?

Children and young people are particularly hard hit by this complex overall situation. They not only experience the fear and anxiety of the adults around them, but also have their own fears about their own future. In addition, they now experience social isolation, and many also domestic violence. Existing hot- lines and child and adolescent psychiatry centres are increasingly overburdened.

In view of these facts, it is understandable that society has become increasingly polarised into those who affirm, justify and support the previous Corona policy and a growing number of citizens who are less and less able to do so and are rebelling against it for a wide variety of reasons. Disputes and conflicts in families, neighbourhoods or at the workplace are the result. Experiencing this potential for conflict, but also the tabooing of the topic for the sake of social peace, has motivated us to look at the different ways of thinking, some of which clash hard, leading to the different positions. For, depending on which view someone has, they back it up with the facts that go with it, and the possibility of mutual understanding is jeopardised.

However, if one can understand the other's way of thinking and allow oneself the search for solutions that do justice to both sides then tolerance and social peace have a chance, with the motivation to engage together and find creative solutions in the face of stressful conflicts. Five of these thought approaches, which have especially contributed with their consequential arguments to the polarization are presented below. Our memorandum is dedicated to the goal of understanding these thought approaches and thereby contributing to a constructive dialogue.

1. What kind of thinking underlies the globally coordinated measures to combat the pandemic?

It is the reductionist way of modern natural science. It assumes the COVID- 19 is a severe, contagious viral disease - not comparable to seasonal flu. Terrifying images of severe cases with fatal consequences and many coffins have etched themselves into the memory of billions of people.

The approach of government officials and the WHO resulting from this insight is clear: the virus must be combated at all costs. In addition, the reasoning makes sense: the health care system would quickly become overburdened and incapable of accommodating all the sick if the pandemic were given free reign. People with pre-existing conditions and of advanced age are particularly at risk, and they need special protection.

The consequence of this way of thinking is to do everything

possible to break the chains of infection, to prevent the severe cases, and to prepare the population for the mass vaccination that will save it. This way of looking at things is consistent, with the 7-day incidence serving as the uniform basis of measurement. Clear figures and facts built on statistical evidence determine the procedure. One could be satisfied with that!

Painful personal, social, cultural and economic collateral damage, however, clearly indicate the extent to which living conditions suffer from this one-sided approach. Especially since impressive current figures from the German Robert Koch Institute (RKI) and World Health Organisation (WHO), show that about 20% or more of the positively tested persons are symptom-free, and the majority of the remaining almost 80% infected show only mild to moderate symptoms. From this point of view, it seems essential to include further points of view and to stimulate a discussion on how these can be combined in such a way that more life-friendly options can become effective.

2. The salutogenic thinking approach asks: Why don't all infected people get sick and of those who do get sick, why don't they all get seriously ill? What keeps people healthy?

Understanding health requires a more complex way of thinking. Health is the unstable equilibrium between the factors that can damage the organism and the regenerative possibilities and resistance forces, which we summarise under the term immunocompetence. Following this way of thinking, the virus is not the only cause of the pandemic - the susceptibility of the organism is another. However, it depends on this susceptibility whether symptoms of disease can develop or not. This fact is also reflected in the infection figures of the WHO (as of 18 August, 2021):

Globally, on the whole earth live 7.87 billion people
Of those tested positive so far: 207,784,507 = 1.58%
Of those tested positive, deceased: 4,370,424 = 2.10% CFR
(=case-fatality rate - by current usage of the term).

Comparing Germany:
Population: 83 million
Tested positive: 3,827,051
Of which died: 91,899 = 2.4%

Comparing UK:
Population: 68 million
Tested positive: 6,295,617
Of which died: 130,979 = 2.1%

Comparing USA:
Population: 333 million
Tested positive: 36,547,639
Of which died: 616,711 = 1.7%

These numbers indicate that on 18 August, 2021, of the world's 7.87 billion people so far 207.8 million have been reported Corona positive and that of those reported positive 2.1% have died (CFR). In Germany, on the same day, the WHO reported a total of 3.83 million people tested Corona positive with PCR test of a total population of 83 million. Of these 2.4% died of or with Corona (CFR). At the same time, it is known that up to now 89% of the deceased in Germany were over 70 years of age and most of them had pre-existing conditions. In the UK it is 82% deaths over 70, *and 97.7% over 50.* These factors indicate an age-related decline in immunocompetence.

This means that the more robust the immune system is and the associated defence situation of the body, the lower the risk of falling ill. In view of these figures, it is understandable that many citizens and experts feel that the government's pandemic regime is disproportionate and ask, for example: Why is there no investment in the healthcare system and in the training of additional nursing and specialist staff? What can be done in terms of health policy so that hospitals are not primarily run for profit but are patient- oriented and equipped for a pandemic? Why not protect the risk groups at a high level, provide high- quality protective clothing for visitors in senior citizens' and nursing homes with quality-tested FFP2 mask protection?

Why are procedures not developed for real risk assessment on-site, i.e. in the actual situations, in the companies, in kindergartens and schools together with those involved, which not only take into account the potential fact that the virus can theoretically affect anyone, but also reckon with the much greater probability that most people will remain healthy? Especially children and adolescents, where severe courses of complications are extremely rare?

3. The psychoimmunological thought approach: What does the fear of illness and death do to us? And what gives us courage?

Already during the first lockdown, a commentary by Dieter Fuchs in the Stuttgarter Zeitung of April 17, 2020, stated, ' 11.4 million families with young children will be forced to somehow organise gainful employment, learning and childcare, in extensive isolation from other people who could help

(...) Their basic rights to education, freedom of movement and social exchange will be ignored. A society that places this burden on parents and children for months at a time will pay a heavy price.'

Since then, the warning voices have increased exponentially. But adults are also paying a high price. Depression increases, chronic diseases worsen. Fear of illness and death, worries about one's own existence, one's job, financial survival or having fewer good educational opportunities - all of this weighs on the mind. What can you do to counteract this?

Why don't the media also highlight what can give courage and what strengthens the immune system in parallel with the daily infection and death figures?[2] Considering that over 90% of Covid deaths are with people with other serious underlying health conditions, why is the only emphasis on vaccination and not on what we can do to improve and maintain health? [3]

At the beginning of the second pandemic wave in the fall, for example, intensive care physician and internist Harald Mattes,

---

[2]   In the UK, emergency powers granted during the Covid crisis, as in war-time, put restrictions on media reporting (see Ofcom letter of 27 March, 2020, *Important guidance – broadcast content on the Coronavirus*, https://www.ofcom.org.uk/__data/assets/pdf_file/0018/205713/annex-a-important-guidance-broadcast-content-on-coronavirus,-27-march-2020.pdf)

[3]   There are also now many reports and studies appearing acknowledging an initial underestimation of what our immune response is capable of in response to Covid, especially with regard to Covid variants. See for instance https://corona-transition.org/israel-verzeichnet-die-hochste-infektionsrate-der-welt or https://www.science.org/news/2021/08/having-sars-cov-2-once-confers-much-greater-immunity-vaccine-vaccination-remains-vital. From the *Science* report: *'"We continue to underestimate the importance of natural infection immunity ... especially when [infection] is recent," says Eric Topol, a physician-scientist at Scripps Research.'* Such findings as well as research on alternate treatments and prevention need to be able to be discussed openly and would help allay fears.

professor at Berlin's Charité and leading physician at Havel-höhe Hospital, called for a shift away from crisis management toward 'risk-stratified action'. Don't we need round tables where such proposals are discussed and then the possibility of practically implementing creative proposals under controlled conditions? How do you strengthen the citizens' own responsibility for their health?

Health and resilience research in the 1970s and 1980s, as well as psychoneuroimmunological research, have in any case amply demonstrated the extent to which negative feelings such as stress, fear, insecurity, powerlessness, persistent worry and despair impair and even damage the immune system. Whereas positive feelings such as courage, hope, confidence, trust, closeness and security strengthen it. Last but not least, it is well known how prayer and meditation can awaken and stabilise positive feelings, especially in times of crisis.

4. The Grassroots Democratic Thinking Approach: Autonomy, Participation and Co-Responsibility

When the well-known American computer expert Josef Weizenbaum visited Germany for lectures and interviews in the "George Orwell" year 1984, he was also asked whether the computer would bring the surveillance state. He could only confirm this and reported that his research and development work had been and is still fully financed by the US Department of Defense. However, he then immediately made it clear (the interview was published in 1984 under the title "Course for the Iceberg") that if the surveillance state were to come, it would not be the fault of the computer, *but of the people who did not defend their freedom.* Hitler and Stalin had demonstrated that surveillance states were not dependent on computers.

Democratic systems, in order to remain functional, need on the one hand the "allure of freedom" (Novalis), on the other hand the joy of dialogue at round tables with those who think differently, in citizens' forums and a fair culture of debate. What conditions are needed in education and training so that such skills can develop?

This question has been explored by education experts like Gerald Hüther for a long time. In his book "Dignity," he calls for an education that helps children and young people to develop an awareness of human dignity and freedom. But how can this be achieved if prescribed norms and regulations tend to increase rather than decrease? Not to mention the additional pressure on children and young people to adapt to the pandemic conditions. It is obvious that a great deal of sensitivity and willingness to talk is necessary in order to agree on a risk-stratified action for the kindergarten and everyday school life among the responsible educators, parents and authorities. Every on-site effort in this regard is all the more worthwhile as school time is precious development time!

5. The Spiritual Thinking Approach and Worldview Issues

Anthroposophy, founded by Rudolf Steiner, was banned at the time of National Socialism, and when the Second World War was over it accomplished significant achievements in the fields of agriculture, medicine, therapeutic education and pedagogy as well as social economic forms - not only in Germany but also worldwide. Even though these achievements are respected and recognised, their "spiritual superstructure", that is, the spiritual way of thinking (called spiritual science by Steiner), is viewed rather with a lack of understanding, questioning why this should be necessary in order to bring about such achievements.

Of course, in the prevailing materialistic-scientific way of thinking there is no place for a science of the spirit as presented in Anthroposophy or other spiritual directions or philosophies. But it is - de facto - not a matter of indifference whether in our own thinking and acting we imagine the human being within a broader spiritual superstructure or not. In other words, it matters what conception of the human being we have in our thinking. Depending on our way of thinking and the conception we have of the human being, the answers to the question of the meaning of life differ. The way we deal with illness and death and the possibility of a spiritual pre-existence and post-existence are also influenced by this. To develop respect and tolerance for this is the core of a humanistic culture.

In view of this fact, it is all the more important to strive for mutual understanding and tolerance of other ways of thinking and seeing things. The best possible compromise for each situation can then be found through negotiation - in accordance with this very fitting saying: Those who want to, find ways - those who don't, find excuses.

Conclusion

The five approaches discussed here are intended as a plea to allow for more interdisciplinary and different ways of looking at the pandemic. Life is a complex process and so is what serves it. Moreover, a development towards freedom and dignity cannot be had without risk. By complementing each other's ways of thinking and the resulting options for action, and by putting claims to sole responsibility into perspective, it is easier to do justice to life in all its complexity. As necessary as a political framework is to contain the pandemic, it is also essential to encourage the population to take personal and shared responsibility and to assess risks realistically in each situation as it presents itself.

About the author

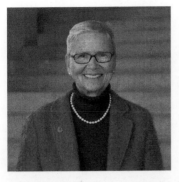

Dr. Michael Glöckler studied German and history with a teaching qualification in Freiburg and Heidelberg, followed by studying medicine in Tübingen and Marburg. She trained as a paediatrician at the Herdecke Community Hospital and the Bochum University Children's Clinic. Until 1987 she worked in the children's outpatient clinic at the Herdecke Community Hospital and as a school doctor at the Rudolf Steiner School in Witten.

From 1988 to 2016 Dr. Glöckler served as head of the Medical Section at the Goetheanum in Dornach, Switzerland. She was Co-founder of the Alliance for Childhood and the European Alliance of Applied Anthroposophy (ELIANT). She lectures and leads training courses internationally for anthroposophic medicine and health-promoting education.

Her books include: *Education for the Future: How to nurture health and human potential*; *A Waldorf Guide to Children's Health* (together with Wolfgang Goebel and Karin Michael); *The Dignity of the Young Child. Care and Training for the First Three Years* (together with Claudia Grah-Wittich); *A Healing Education: How can Waldorf Education Meet the Needs of Children*; *Education as Preventive Medicine: A Salutogenic Approach*; *Leadership Questions and Forms of Working in the Anthroposophic Medical Movement*; *Truth, Beauty and Goodness – the future of education, healing arts and Health care*; *What is Anthroposophic Medicine?*; *Medicine at the Threshold*; *Meditations on Heart-Activity*; and many further publications.

Branko Furst, MD, FFARCSI (author of the Foreword) - is a graduate of the University of Ljubljana School of Medicine, Slovenia and completed residency in anesthesiology at the Queen Alexandra Hospital in Portsmouth and at the Middlesex Hospitals in London, UK. In 1987 he joined the faculty at the Department of Anesthesiology at Texas Tech University Medical School in El Paso, TX. Currently he is Professor of Anesthesiology at Albany Medical College, Albany, NY and divides his time between clinical practice, research, and resident teaching. He has lectured on the integrative model of circulation nationally and internationally. He is author of the book, *The Heart and Circulation: An Integrative Model*, currently in second edition (Springer Verlag), which has been translated into German under the title, *Autonomie der Blutbewegung* [Autonomous movement of the blood], Salumed Verlag.

Andreas Neider, MA (co-author of the Appendix) studied philosophy, ethnology, history and politics. His work has spanned lecturing, publishing and, since 2002, he has been director of the German cultural agency, 'Von Mensch zu Mensch'. He is author of *Denken mit dem Herzen: Wie wir unsere Gedanken aus dem Kopf befreien können* [Thinking with the heart: how we can free our thoughts from the head]; co-author of *Corona - Eine Krise und ihre Bewältigung* [Corona - a crisis and how we can deal with it]; co-author of *Corona und die Überwindung der Getrenntheit* [Corona and overcoming separation], and numerous other German language publications.

93

Further titles by InterActions

https://interactions360.org

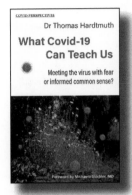

WHAT COVID-19 CAN TEACH US
Meeting the virus with fear or informed common sense?

by Thomas Hardtmuth, MD.
Foreword by Michaela Glöckler, MD.

2021. ISBN 978-0-9528364-4-5
94 pages, UK £7.50, USA $12

First in the InterActions Covid Perspectives series, Dr Hardtmuth provides a detailed, highly readable analysis of the multi-dimensional Corona crisis, including an in-depth view of our immune system resilience with the latest science recognising viruses not as 'enemies' but as vital for human evolution and health. This holistic perspective suggests new approaches not only for treatment but also prevention. He examines further details around the Covid pandemic including the PCR test reliability, risks and benefits of vaccination, and fear's negative effect on immunity.

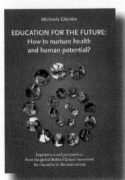

EDUCATION FOR THE FUTURE:
How to nurture health and human potential?

by Michaela Glöckler, MD.

2020. ISBN 978-0-9528364-3-8
UK £19.99   USA $28
248 pages. Pb, colour photos and illustrations.

Education for the Future is a plea for radically aligning upbringing and education with what is needed for the healthy development and well-being of children and adolescents. A unique contribution of Dr Glöckler is a year-by-year examination of human biological development and how this relates to soul-spiritual development, which in turn has a direct bearing on the needs of the child within upbringing and education. A treasure chest of information and insights for educators, parents, carers and therapists.

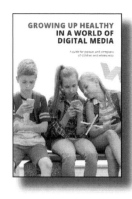

GROWING UP HEALTHY IN A WORLD OF DIGITAL MEDIA
A guide for parents and caregivers of children and adolescents.

Written by specialists from 15 organisations concerned with media and childhood development. Introduction by Dr Michaela Glöckler.

2019. ISBN 9780 9528364 14, UK £10, 160 pages, sewn pb, colour illustrations and photos.

With increased screen use from Covid epidemic restrictions, this new guide is more relevant than ever. It explains child development considerations, noting dangers of inappropriate use and giving practical advice for a positive *age appropriate* use of digital media. It integrates a holistic approach, with consideration of physical, emotional and mental development of children. Easy to read. *An essential guide.*

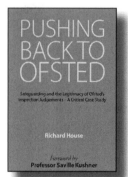

PUSHING BACK TO OFSTED
Safeguarding and the legitimacy of Ofsted's inspection judgements - a critical case study

by Richard House, PhD.
Foreword by Prof. Saville Kushner.
2020, ISBN 978-0-9528364-2-1,
128 pages. Pb. UK £10.99

'Ofsted' (Office for Standards in Education) in England is considered to be one of the harshest school inspectorates in the world. Dr House wrote this book following the closure of several Waldorf schools in the UK due to Ofsted inspections. He sets out in relentless detail the shortcomings and prejudices of the Ofsted report for one of those schools, as an example for how a state's one-size-fits-all approach can perpetuate a kind of violence on educational creativity and freedoms. It is a helpful study for schools facing intense state scrutiny and judgement. *"This analysis... is an uncomfortable but necessary challenge to current educational orthodoxies."* Dr. Rowan Williams, former Archbishop of Canterbury.

New InterActions titles
for publication autumn/winter 2021

(Provisional details)

LIMITS TO MEDICAL SCIENCE:
'Revolutionary' Conversations.

edited by Richard House, PhD

Interviews with medical professionals, philosophers, psychologists and researchers. Expected publication date, late autumn/winter 2021.

BEING HUMAN IN THE HERE AND NOW:
Conversations with the soul of my sister Ajra

(provisional title)

by Ana Pogacnik

Conversations with the soul of her parted sister reveal insights into our human existence, on earth and in life after life, in our challenges including the grave spiritual consequences of Corona vaccinations, and in the hopes for our future.
Translated from the German. Publication late Autumn 2021.

*Further in the **Covid Perspectives** series –*
CORONA AND THE RIDDLE OF IMMUNITY

edited by Andreas Neider and Michaela Glöckler

Contributions from medical, biological, educational, sociological and philosophical perspectives. Translated from the German. Expected publication date, late autumn/winter 2021-22.

VACCINATING THE WORLD?
Critical perspectives, informed 'hesitancy'
by Richard House, PhD

A new study of the mass-vaccination phenomenon, including an extensive literature review and Philosophy of Science perspectives on the metaphysics underpinning the vaccination worldview. Expected publication date, late autumn/winter 2021.

For further details, when available, see our website
https://interactions360.org/our-books/